THESE
VITAL
SIGNS

THESE VITAL SIGNS

A DOCTOR'S NOTES ON
LIFE AND LOSS IN TWEETS

SAYED TABATABAI

HARPER

An Imprint of HarperCollinsPublishers

HarperCollins books may be purchased for educational, business, or sales promotional use. For information, please email the Special Markets Department at SPsales@harpercollins.com.

FIRST EDITION

Library of Congress Cataloging-in-Publication Data has been applied for.

23 24 25 26 27 LBC 5 4 3 2 1

FOR ALL THE PEOPLE WHO FOLLOWED ME ON TWITTER
AND SUPPORTED MY WRITING.
WITHOUT YOU, THIS BOOK WOULDN'T EXIST.

AND FOR MY FAMILY.
ALL THE GOOD IN ME,
FLOWS FROM THEM.

Contents

Preface

It is the summer of 1991 and I am facing off against my most determined foe: the blank page. I'm ten years old, and I have to write a story for a holiday assignment. My grandmother sits on the couch behind me, as I lie on my belly on the floor, idly doodling in the margins of my notebook. I can hear the rhythmic hiss of her oxygen tank. She has idiopathic pulmonary fibrosis, a condition I'm too young to comprehend. Many years later I will understand and write about her illness.

She watches me and smiles. Her voice is weak but still strong enough to catch my ear. "If you don't know where to start writing, start at the beginning."

I answer the way I usually answer anyone at this age, with a question: "How do I know where the beginning is?"

She laughs. "The beginning is where your mind goes to first, when you close your eyes."

Thirty years later, as I sit in front of my laptop, I close my eyes and let my mind wander. I see snow falling gently from cloudy skies and slowly accumulating on a hospital room windowsill.

If my story is to begin anywhere, let it be at the very beginning. I am born in 1980, on a snowy Christmas day, in Baltimore, Maryland. My father is an engineer who is pursuing an MBA at the University of Maryland in College Park at the time. My mother is a teacher who will someday win awards for her work. The nurse brings me out to my family for the first time in a little red stocking. Everyone is overjoyed. I am the answer to many prayers, as I am told years later.

After graduating from the University of Maryland, my father gets a job with an international construction conglomerate. His engineering and business background, along with his coolheaded leadership style and natural charisma, make him a popular man. He is assigned to larger and larger projects in different countries. My childhood is spent crisscrossing the world.

The earliest memory I have is of a fountain, arching high into the sky. So high, in fact, that when I look up at it, I'm convinced it's going to topple over onto me. It is an optical illusion, but it terrifies me. I'm sitting on my father's shoulders, and he laughs as I squirm anxiously. We are in the courtyard of some famous Austrian palace. But I can't see the beauty. I can't see past my own fear.

There are some things in life that seem so insurmountable they threaten to crush us. As a child, for me, it is the fountain. Years later, as I exit a subway station in New York City on my way to a residency interview, the looming skyscrapers make me queasy. They seem to threaten to topple over when I look up at them, so I force my gaze down at the pavement and try to quell the rising anxiety within me. Old phobias. The past is never far.

I reach the hospital I'm interviewing at for an internal medicine residency position. These interviews are carefully structured and I find myself loathing their artifice. Everyone tells me all the tricks interviewers use to weed out applicants. I have no time for tricks or traps. I bludgeon my way through with brutal honesty.

"What do you enjoy doing in your free time?"

"I write."

"Oh? What kind of writing?"

"All sorts of writing. I write in a journal, on a blog, in a—"

"So personal writing. Not medical journals."

"No, not medical journals."

Years later, I will be published in medical journals. But right now it seems like a gaping hole in my résumé. My written words are valued only by me.

In 2019, I begin to experiment with writing on Twitter. The character limit provides me with a spark in my writing that I have been lacking for years. A way to bring form and structure, a challenge, a forced paring down of my verbiage. I discover that writing on Twitter has its own rhythms and they come naturally to me.

At first, I write as a kidney doctor giving advice. This is recommended to me, to grow my "brand." It is a miserable experience, full of words but bereft of meaning. I decide to leave that voice behind and use my own. Instead of being the physician tweeter,

I begin writing as a human being, who just happens to be a physician.

Medicine becomes the lens through which I focus in on life, from the largest sweeping themes to the minutiae that make us who we are. I don't expect my ramblings to resonate with anyone. Every time I click "tweet" I feel like I am sending them into a void from which no response will ever come. But slowly the response begins to build. When the likes start spiraling into the thousands, it feels for me both deeply gratifying as a writer and terrifying as an introvert. Dopamine and disorientation.

I quickly find that my writing is resonating intensely with a wide variety of people. Perhaps because I speak the language of human emotion and loss as opposed to just clinical data, I am inadvertently helping to fill in the blind spots in modern scientific communication from other members of my profession. Whatever it is, it gives me an unexpected platform and the support of thousands of strangers I'll never meet.

I consider myself extremely fortunate to have had this avenue of self-expression. I can't imagine my world without it. Three years later, I've poured my heart and soul into my writing on Twitter. I've managed to make friends and establish myself on a tiny island in the endless ocean of tweets that are generated every day. I've written more than a hundred stories and honed my craft in this strange new medium of "tweetistry." For years people have been asking me for a compilation of these stories, something that would save them time and provide a bit of background to the tales.

It is in this spirit that this book is being written, for the people who have encouraged me, shown me such warmth and such love. Without them I would never have kept writing as I did. It is a collection of short stories, and the stories behind them. I hope this endeavor brings you happiness and fulfillment, as it has done so for me, a thousand times over.

The medical stories I write involve characters that are composites of patients I have encountered over the past almost twenty years of practicing medicine in four different states across America. Names are created and story details are altered to protect privacy, and often are blended from multiple patients—except for my biographical stories; those are as they are.

Thank you for taking these journeys with me.

PART I

Beginnings

There are times in your life when you discover something new about someone that you never expected to find. Sometimes the discoveries are unpleasant, sometimes they're remarkable, but whatever they are, they often cast a new light on the person. You might have thought you knew the person well and then discover that you had no idea what depths they carried within them. So it was with my paternal grandfather.

Throughout my life I knew my grandfather as a military man, rigid and upright, regimented and disciplined. He had reached the rank of brigadier general in the army and retired to live a quiet life with his wife, spending time with his many children and grandchildren when they visited. He would wake up before anyone else in the house, get the newspaper from the porch, and sit down at the table in the kitchen. As we all slept, he would read through the newspaper thoroughly, sipping on a cup of tea and slowly, leisurely, peeling an apple to eat a slice at a time.

I had heard through my parents that my grandfather enjoyed poetry. Our culture places a high value on the ability to recite intricate and beautiful prose. I knew that he went to get-togethers where poetry recitation was the main attraction. What I didn't know was that my grandfather was an accomplished poet. He wrote verses upon verses of achingly beautiful poetry, and the intensity and beauty of his work only increased after the tragic death of his beloved wife, my grandmother. He wrote his poetry with a fervor, as if it might spare his soul, at least temporarily, from the grief of her passing.

It was only after he died that I discovered the depth and breadth of my grandfather's love for poetry. A posthumous compilation of his writing was published, and I remember holding the book in my hands and running my fingertips along the paper, feeling its texture.

He wrote in his native language that wasn't my own, but I listened to people explain his work and felt tears stinging my eyes. My whole life I have felt the urge to write, since I was a child writing my own adventure stories, through the journals I kept throughout my medical education, to these words I'm typing now. If only I had known that my grandfather wrote as much as he recited. How I wish I could talk to him still.

Was he happy with what he wrote? Were words left unsaid? Even if you've said everything you meant to say, there always remains a small crack through which new light filters through. Light from another sunrise, another tomorrow.

Humsafar

He walks through the cemetery gates early in the morning. His footsteps are slowed by age and unsteadiness.

He is there almost every day, and the groundskeepers recognize him now.

"The old man who writes" they call him.

And "the old man who cries."

He is my grandfather.

◇◇◇

As he makes his way to his usual spot, he has a folding chair under one arm and holds a bouquet of flowers under the other.

He tries to hold himself firmly upright, back straight, even though arthritis has set in.

He used to be a brigadier general.
Old habits die hard.

◇◇◇

Reaching his destination, his eyes fill with tears for a moment or two, as they always do.

"Hello, love, my dearest friend."

He reaches down and gently rests a hand on her tombstone, whispering a prayer. Then he sets up the folding chair.

◇◇◇

She was the youngest daughter in an aristocratic family, fiercely independent, and determinedly horse riding while the rest of her four sisters were married off one by one.

Her father was a nawab, a distinguished scholar, and an acclaimed poet.

They lived on a palatial estate.

◇◇◇

He was one of five brothers and one sister. His family was learned. They didn't have much money, but they had their education, and this brought them respect.

He was rakishly handsome, with an offhand charm that won him many friends. A favorite among his military peers.

◇◇◇

Those were different times, in a different culture, and there was no courtship then.

The women in the families connected with one another, and matchmaking occurred in an intricately layered web of acquaintances.

My grandparents met for the first time on their wedding day.

◇◇◇

Right away, theirs was a true match.

She had never gone to school but had been taught by tutors who came to her house every day. She spoke four languages fluently.

Every time he quoted her a romantic verse, she would quote him back its reply, and then the next verses too.

◇◇◇

India, in those days, was in the process of a great upheaval.

The end of colonial British rule, and the breaking apart of society along religious and cultural fault lines, led to the splintering of families and a bloody period of rebirth.

Change came for everyone.

My grandparents found refuge and solace in each other. The strains on their relationship, as the world around them frayed and cracked, only brought them closer together.

"Humsafar," like so many foreign words, loses much of its meaning in translation.

"Traveling companion."

◇◇◇

But humsafar is more than just a traveling companion.

Life is a journey, a slingshot trajectory between two great unknowns

A flickering transition between two infinities.

Humsafar means I will journey with you. I will believe in you.

I will remain by your side.

The years pass, on this journey.

They have four children. Two boys and two girls. My father is the second oldest.

Education is their mantra. My father is an engineer, one sister is a teacher, the other is a doctor, and the youngest son an army major and then a teacher.

◇◇◇

There are not enough pages in the world for me to write of the depths and breadths of a life well lived, but inevitably there is the end.

If life teaches us anything, it is a bittersweet lesson in letting go.

My grandmother dies of breast cancer in 1998.

His beloved humsafar is gone.

◇◇◇

The light goes out in my grandfather's eyes after that.

His doctors say he has a broken heart, cardiomyopathy, and he eventually goes into kidney failure and needs to start dialysis. He is dying.

But there is one area in which he flourishes.

His secret.

His poetry.

He writes under a pen name: Raaz.

It means "a secret."

As he sits by her grave, on his little folding chair, he writes, and he weeps.

After his humsafar leaves him, he writes achingly beautiful verses, elegies, inspired by a love that brings him all the words he seeks.

◇◇◇

When he gets up to leave, he lays the flowers by her headstone and then places several on the graves on either side of hers.

He never knew these people, but they are his beloved's neighbors now.

He has always been kind to his neighbors.

◇◇◇

He finally leaves this world for a long-awaited reunion, in January of 2001.

At his funeral I am overwhelmed by how many people are there, how many have flown in from other countries to be there, how many lives he has touched.

I hear my grandfather's poetry praised repeatedly.

◇◇◇

To this day, I cannot read or understand his poetry. There is a language barrier I cannot overcome, yet. The translations I've read remain frustratingly inadequate.

It is perhaps one last irony. That the "secret" should remain hidden from me, when I seek it the most.

◇◇◇

And now here I am. Walking a path that seems to reach out to me from the past.

Echoes of a life lived before mine.

Healing kidneys for a living.

Chasing the "secret" in my spare time.

Perhaps one day

someday

◇◇◇

I'll find it.

In His Footsteps

The young doctor wonders how he got here, staring down the cold barrel of a gun.

The year is 1960, and he has a wife and little children.

The man with the gun tells him to change the autopsy report or else.

The young doctor takes a deep breath, then exhales slowly.

"No."

◇◇◇

But stories don't begin at the end, do they?

Let's go back to the beginning.

The year is 1926.

A boy is born into a large family in a village near Batala, in Punjab, India. His family lives in poverty, as farmers.

He is born with no hope and no future beyond his village.

◇◇◇

One day, as he is helping his brothers with farm work, he realizes that unless he tries to change it, his life and the lives of his family will be caught up in an endless cycle of poverty.

He is eight when this realization comes.

This boy doesn't know it yet, but he has a great gift. The power of insight, and compassion.

The gift of empathy.

He knows in his heart that he can't just save himself and his family from this impoverished life. He must help others too.

His path to salvation?

Education.

◇◇◇

He tells his two best friends his plan.

He is too poor to go to school, but he has persuaded someone to help teach them to read.

He can't afford books, but together the three best friends can buy one book, and they tear it into three parts.

Hope flares brilliantly to life.

◇◇◇

Working during the day, studying during the night, the three friends slowly and painstakingly build up their most precious treasure: knowledge.

They read book after book, one third at a time.

They quiz one another, as they fall asleep, exhausted, sore, often hungry.

Finally, they reach a milestone. They are ready to take the exams for the schools in the big city nearby.

They can't pay for an education, but if their scores are high enough, they can win scholarships.

Their families pray for them, and the three boys journey to the city.

◇◇◇

All three boys win scholarships. The school staff is amazed; nobody from the farmlands has ever been admitted.

The gifted boy, the empath, is more determined than ever now.

He is convinced that fate has brought him here for a reason.

He chooses to pursue medicine.

◇◇◇

1947 comes, and the boy is now a young man.

During the Partition, he migrates to the newly formed Pakistan and becomes one of the doctors in the first-ever Pakistani medical school class.

He is a gifted clinician, beloved by his colleagues, his patients, and his community.

◇◇◇

For the first time in his life, he is not anxiously trying to scrape together enough money for food, books, everything.

He uses his new wealth to educate his family in the village and pull as many of the people in his community out of poverty as he can.

He makes this his life's mission.

◇◇◇

The years pass, and he gets married to a wonderful woman.

One day, many decades after their wedding day, she will be lying in a hospital bed, delirious, as her lungs fail from idiopathic pulmonary fibrosis. Her son will hold her hand.

◇◇◇

They have three children in the years ahead. Two boys and one girl.

The little girl will have her own children someday: my sister and me.

The young doctor is my maternal grandfather.

◇◇◇

And the day finally comes in 1960 when he faces a gun and a demand he cannot accept.

◇◇◇

A powerful man has committed a murder. He has shot someone in cold blood. The doctor performing the autopsy is my grandfather.

His autopsy report will condemn the powerful man by the means and nature of the wounds.

The powerful man has hired an assassin.

My grandfather faces that assassin with a look of sadness. He knows what the man with the gun wants, but he can never compromise on his principles.

To do so would betray everything he is. He must do the right thing.

He is told at gunpoint to change his report.

He says no.

The assassin begins to pull the trigger.

◇◇◇

But fate isn't done with my grandfather yet.

Perhaps it's the sight of the young man making a last stand for his principles.

Perhaps it's the photo of his young family on his desk.

The assassin doesn't shoot.

Instead, he flees.

◇◇◇

My grandfather is wise enough to realize that sooner or later another man with a gun will come for him.

He takes his family into hiding. But he still shows up in court to testify on his autopsy findings.

That whole day his entire family prays for his survival.

It works.

◇◇◇

But my grandfather is understandably deeply shaken by the experience. He decides to leave Pakistan with his young family.

A United Nations mission is recruiting physicians to work in Africa.

My grandfather journeys to Maiduguri, in northeastern Nigeria, and sets up a clinic.

◇◇◇

Committed to compassionate care, he becomes well known for his kindness, and treats everyone regardless of their ability to pay.

He continues to cherish education and gets his diploma in tropical medicine and hygiene from the Royal College of Physicians in London.

◇◇◇

My own memories of him, from my early childhood, are hazy.

Two, in particular, stand out.

One, where he is greeting me and my parents at the airport. He reaches to embrace me, and I hide behind my dad's legs feeling overwhelmed with shyness.

I remember his kind smile.

◇◇◇

The second, and last, memory is more concrete. It takes place in 1985.

I am five years old at the time.

My mother receives a phone call in the middle of the night. She is pregnant with my sister.

Her cry of anguish awakens me.

I watch her sob and start to cry myself.

◇◇◇

My grandfather's death is sudden, unexpected. A heart attack, they say.

I don't realize the depths of this loss until much later in life.

As I get older, people tell me I look like him. I smile like him. I have his nature.

I owe everything to his realization when he was eight.

Without knowing it, I have walked in his shadow my whole life. Hoping to live up to the standards set by a person I'll never get to know, that everyone loved so much.

One grandfather a warrior poet, one grandfather an empathic healer.

PART II

The Lessons

The stories in this part concern the journey I took toward medicine. Though I may have inherited the urge to write from my paternal grandfather, that doesn't necessarily mean I inherited his reasons too. Where I began writing in earnest was in medical school and during my postgraduate medical training, and it was as a means of survival. I realized early on that my medical training would be a crucible in which I was going to be forged.

In this forging, I feared I would lose some essential part of myself. I saw the process of becoming a physician like that of becoming a guitarist: Before you could pluck sharp steel strings you needed your fingertips to grow calluses. Callused skin would be numb to the pain and then you could make music. But I was afraid that by growing numb, I would lose the raw, sensitive part of me that cared so deeply about why all of this mattered.

The stories concerning my medical education in this part are not focused on the minutiae of the process itself. Instead, like most of the stories in this book, they focus on the broader themes and the humanity within a process that can seem to take away as much as it gives to those willing to brave it.

Many of the deepest and most lasting lessons I've learned in medicine haven't been the dramatic ones that announce themselves with fanfare and great expectations. No, the lasting lessons have come in the quiet moments. The subtle and human moments that make us who we are, and in doing so, tell our stories. These moments don't always present themselves in obvious ways. You must be patient and willing to listen. You have to take the time and make the space.

The Old Surgeon

The surgeon's hand is visibly trembling.

The scalpel's blade glints as it catches the light.

I'm a medical student, scrubbed in on the case. I'm not going into surgery, I know that. I'm here for him.

He glances at me and notices that I'm holding my breath.

He grins.

"Relax."

◇◇◇

My medical school experience so far has been a lengthy gestation in the womb of the lecture hall.

I have soaked in more words than I ever thought I could.
Books and lectures. I have learned anatomy, and physiology, and pathology, and more.

I know so much.

I know nothing.

◇◇◇

My first inkling of just how vast the distance is from where I am to where I want to be is in the dissection lab. The second is with the standardized patient encounters.

The dawning realization hits me: I have been learning to ride a bike by reading about it.

◇◇◇

When I get the opportunity to rotate with practicing doctors in the community, I make a decision.

They say you should work with docs in a field you're interested in. But I want to work with the "best" clinicians, no matter what their field.

I need to learn the art of this.

◇◇◇

And so the old surgeon was recommended to me by almost everyone I spoke to.

"A doctor's doctor," they tell me. Whatever that means.

I call him "the old surgeon" because that's what he calls himself. He's on the verge of retirement.

I am one of his last students.

◇◇◇

The day I first meet him, he comes out to the lobby to greet me and takes me back into his office.

He treats me like an old friend he is seeing again after a long time.

I'm surprised. I don't know what I was expecting, but it wasn't this.

His smile is contagious.

◇◇◇

The office is filled with books, medical and otherwise, and the walls are covered with photographs. Friends, family, patients perhaps?

He tells me I am here to learn and he will do his best to teach me. That no question is off-limits, and that no answer will be ridiculed.

◇◇◇

His eyebrows are bushy and seem accentuated by his baldness. Like giant caterpillars wiggling expressively.

I can't help but smile.

As we get ready to go to the hospital to do some rounding, he tells me that he does have one rule for me to abide by.

◇◇◇

"Treat everyone you meet with respect and kindness. Especially the patients."

He pauses for a moment, looking back at me over his shoulder, as if making sure he doesn't lose me.

"Especially them, okay?"

"Okay." I nod, filled with the enthusiastic resolve of the novice.

◇◇◇

As the day progresses, I'm starting to realize why the old surgeon is regarded so highly.

He sits down at the bedsides. He isn't afraid to hold hands if they're offered or accept hugs.

He has a way of making it seem like time is irrelevant when he's focusing on you.

◇◇◇

I notice the small details, soaking them up.

He knows all the nurses' names. The clerical staff. The janitors. The security guards. The transport staff. And he greets everyone.

He even pronounces "Tabatabai" correctly, on the second try.

I realize it's about respect.

◇◇◇

As we round, he teaches me specific things, and also general pearls.

His vast experience has given him perspective. I'm impressed with how often he chooses NOT to operate.

He senses my surprise and explains simply, "Do no harm."

He understands the words better than I do.

◇◇◇

He's sitting with a patient, talking about an upcoming surgery. The patient is understandably anxious.

The old surgeon takes his time, explaining clearly, fielding questions, and answering thoughtfully.

And then he asks the patient about their dog.

The patient is surprised and then tells him the dog's name and how much they love them.

The old surgeon smiles. "I've got two dogs. They're like my kids. They walk me every day." He looks across at me. "Got a dog, Sayed?"

I shake my head.

He grins. "Get one!"

◇◇◇

"All right," the old surgeon says to the patient. "Let's get this surgery done and get you home to your furry friend ASAP. Sound good?"

The patient smiles and nods.

I don't know quite what the surgeon has just done, but I know he did something essential.

Something kind.

◇◇◇

Later on, in the operating room, I realize that the old surgeon has a pretty noticeable resting tremor.

The scalpel trembles as he grips it.

Without realizing I'm doing it, I hold my breath as I watch the shining blade begin to shakily descend.

He notices and grins. "Relax."

◇◇◇

As the surgery progresses, I'm amazed at how the tremor has vanished and how smooth and assured his hands are.

He operates with steady precision and economy of movement.

I don't know much about surgery, but I know enough to appreciate mastery.

◇◇◇

The surgery is a success.

He goes out to the waiting room to inform the family members and is tearfully hugged.

He always introduces me to everyone, and he does so again here. He says I was invaluably helpful, even though I wasn't at all.

I am hugged.

It feels . . . real.

◇◇◇

At the day's end, he asks me if I have any questions.

I have one.

"How did you know that patient had a dog?"

He smiles. "Doggy bone on the keychain, bedside table. There's another lesson, Sayed: Observe!"

I laugh as his bushy eyebrows wiggle to accentuate his point.

◇◇◇

Years later, and students are rotating with me.

I feel the awesome responsibility of trying to impart something meaningful.

I try to draw upon the wisdom of the many incredible teachers I've had along the way.

The students will learn the science.

It's the art that's elusive.

Truth in the Tracings

"How many letters are there in the alphabet?"

I had been expecting a question, just not this one. Damn.

Uhh. Twenty-six. Right?

. . . Right? Argh, this is so simple, but why is it so difficult?

"Twenty-six," I say.

The cardiology fellow who asked me the question grins. "Perhaps."

◇◇◇

Perhaps? What does that mean? I glance at the other house staff, and there are a few nervous shrugs.

The fellow continues. "It might be 26, or it might not. Depends on the language."

Oh, right.

◇◇◇

Medical training tends to create a singularly stressful environment.
You're trying to learn an art and a science, immersed in an entirely new highly technical jargon with thousands of words.

You're trying to figure out what you want to do with your life within this vast world.

And you're trying to make a good impression while doing it. Every time you're asked a question, it may be an opportunity for learning, but it also feels like an opportunity to prove yourself.

A missed question on rounds can hang over your head in ways few things can.

A missed opportunity to shine.

◇◇◇

I'm an intern on the cardiac electrophysiology (EP) rotation. My fellow for the rotation is a tall gentleman with a rumbling baritone and a mind like a steel trap.

He's kind. The quiet sort.

And willing to teach.

I sit before him and his EKGs are spread out on the table.

◇◇◇

EKGs are the heart and soul of this rotation. If you can't read them, you're like a sailor who can't navigate, a scholar who can't read.

I stare at the line tracings. Electrical signals rippling through fibers and muscle.

◇◇◇

The fellow describes the EKGs to me. I've read books on them. Studied them already. But I don't see them, not like he does.

"To be honest, I don't really see the lines anymore. Not like that. I see . . ." He scratches his brow. ". . . the heart. Visualize it, how it's beating."

◇◇◇

I shake my head. "I can't read them like you can."

He nods. "Well, of course. It's experience, isn't it? I've just read several thousand more of these than you. Give it time."

I nod, exhaling deeply.

And we return to studying the EKGs and the secrets between the lines.

◇◇◇

I know that I don't want to go into cardiology, at least not EP. It feels too detached from the human experience. At least to me.

For me, the EKGs are windows to circuitry, not people.

But I study hard, like with every rotation. To add skills, and perhaps understanding.

◇◇◇

But I will never see the EKGs the way the fellow does. The more he explains them, the more I realize we are seeing them in two completely different ways.

◇◇◇

At the end of our impromptu teaching session, I have one last question.

"This morning, why did you ask me about the letters in the alphabet?"

He thinks for a moment. "Because perspective is important. With EKGs. With life."

Finally, I understand.

He smiles and gets up.

◇◇◇

Before he leaves, he turns to ask me one more thing. "How many bones in the body?"

I think for a bit. "Depends on the body?"

He grins. "Good man. Oh, and if the attendings ask you any questions about arrhythmias, the answer is 'reentry' about 99% of the time."

I laugh.

◇◇◇

The next day the EP attendings are having their morning rounds, with the house staff clustered around the table in a reverential hush.

Suddenly one of the attendings points to a tiny squiggle on an EKG and then points at me. "You. What does this mean?"

A chance to shine.

◇◇◇

Before I speak, I glance at the fellow. He gives the smallest of nods, and I smile.

"Reentry," I say.

"Excellent. This is what triggers the aberrant conduction and leads to . . ."

As the attending carries on, I smile, feeling the endorphin rush of an answered question.

◇◇◇

How many letters are in the alphabet?

How many bones are in the body?

I knew a cardiology fellow who saw a beating heart instead of EKGs.

We see not only what we can.

We see what we choose to.

The Invisible Milestones

At some point, your parents picked you up, set you down, and never picked you up again.

I don't know who first said that, but the thought has been lingering with me.

There are invisible milestones we cross every day, unknowingly.

Last times, and first times, for everything.

◇◇◇

The ICU is always deceptively quiet when I enter. The controlled chaos on the battlefields of life and death is contained, one room at a time.

I'm here today to see a case of something I've never seen before.

◇◇◇

I sit down at a workstation and pull up the chart.

There is a discipline to reviewing a chart. The temptation to skim and see what you want to see, to fit your biases, is very strong.

Often important clues are embedded in seemingly trivial details.

Start at the beginning.

◇◇◇

I read through the Emergency Medical Services ambulance note.

911 call for an unresponsive patient. Woman in her 50s. Lethargic, hypotensive, blood pressure in the 90s over 50s.

Tachycardia, heart rate in the 110s. IV access, fluid bolus.

Code 3—lights and sirens.

◇◇◇

On arrival to the emergency department, the patient has wide complex tachycardia, a potentially unstable heart rhythm.

The heart, like any other muscle, contracts based on electrical activity carried along a conduction system.

When things go wrong, we can try to hit reset.

◇◇◇

An electrical charge is applied, a shock.

Cardioversion is an attempt to reset the circuitry and allow the heart's natural pacemaker, the sinus node, to recapture the rhythm.

In this case, it doesn't work.

A second attempt doesn't work either.

Transfer to the ICU.

◇◇◇

An intravenous anti-arrhythmic medication is tried, without success.

At this point the patient's labs reveal liver failure and kidney failure.

She is awake, but drowsy. Lapsing in and out of alertness.

Her heart rate is in the low 110s, and the rhythm remains wide complex.

◇◇◇

On many levels, nephrology is an extremely data-driven specialty.

Before I ever see a patient, I have immersed myself in the world of their data.

Numbers have painted a picture.

I know them on a level of milligrams per deciliter and milliequivalents per liter.

◇◇◇

I know their anions, and their cations. I know their acidity, and their osmolality. I know how well their kidneys are filtering, excreting.

I know all of this. And I know nothing.

Because none of this is who we are.

No more than a building is just the sum of its bricks.

◇◇◇

There always comes a moment in a consultation when you cross that threshold from the abstract to the concrete.

When the numbers become the person.

The data are always a moment in time, anyway. Static and unyielding.

Humans are beautifully imperfect, in constant flux.

◇◇◇

The patient looks ashen. Extremities cold and clammy. She looks at me with glassy eyes. Her urine looks like brown sludge in the catheter.

Blood pressures are marginal. The heart rhythm on the monitor is constantly setting off alarms.

I perform my physical examination.

◇◇◇

She seems to be drifting in and out of clarity as I feel her thready pulse beneath my fingertips.

But suddenly her gaze is clear. She looks right at me, as if seeing me for the first time.

"I'm sick, right?"

I nod. "Yes."

"Am I dying?"

I shake my head. "No, you're not."

◇◇◇

She nods, exhaling. "I wasn't ready for it to be my last time doing things."

And just like that she drifts back into whatever world she came to me from, halfway between the living and the dead.

I finish my exam and step back outside the room.

Her words linger with me.

◇◇◇

How many invisible milestones do we cross every day unknowingly?

A time came when I hugged my grandparents for the last time.

When I played fetch with my old dog Caesar for the last time.

When I left my childhood home, never to return.

Invisible milestones all around us.

◇◇◇

A week later and the patient is laughing and joking with me.

Her recovery was nothing short of remarkable. Heart, kidneys, liver.

Everything.

It's amazing how her personality lights up the world around her. Her smile is warm and kind.

She makes us all smile with her.

Into the Photos

Sometimes it's the things that are right in front of us that we just can't see.

I'm sitting in a patient's room in the ICU.

The patient's family sits with me.

I'm tired.

I drift.

◇◇◇

The patient is an elderly gentleman. He has heart failure and kidney failure, and has developed a bloodstream infection.

I hear the dreaded terms "multi-organ failure" and "septic shock." Words that feel sharp on my tongue.

Jagged.

He is unconscious, sedated on a ventilator.

◇◇◇

In this state he is unknowable, unresponsive, and unreachable.

But his family has put up photographs on his bedside and on one wall of the room.

And through these photos he suddenly becomes vibrantly alive.

I stand up and move closer to the wall, so I can see . . .

◇◇◇

A photo.

The elderly gentleman is much younger. He wears a military uniform and holds himself stiffly upright.

His gaze is on the distance. His chest glitters with medals.

He looks handsome. And somewhat uncomfortable.

I sense the pomp and ceremony aren't his thing.

◇◇◇

A photo.

The elderly gentleman is sitting with friends and family, laughing.

His face is kind. He has many stories to share and tell.

I notice how everyone seems to be smiling at him.

He draws everyone's attention and gives them back happiness in return.

Fair trade.

◇◇◇

A photo.

The elderly gentleman is a young father. His four young children are standing duly at attention in front of him. They're dressed in their finest.

His wife stands beside him. She looks elegant, a silk shawl across her shoulders.

Everyone smiles for the camera.

◇◇◇

A photo.

Black-and-white. From the late '40s, early '50s. The elderly gentleman is a dashing young man, and he's a newlywed.

He's behind the wheel of a car that looks new, with large fins. His wife sits beside him, beaming.

The world is so full of promise.

◇◇◇

A photo.

The elderly man is holding up a grandson, laughing at the chubby baby's bewildered smile.

The baby will grow up to love and respect his grandfather. One day he will look at this photo and smile.

I know this for a fact, because it's me in the photo.

◇◇◇

I reach out to run my fingertips along the photo.

The elderly gentleman is actually my grandfather.

The patient's family is actually my own.

He is unresponsive and unreachable. But he is still every bit a person and human being.

And I love him.

◇◇◇

A photo.

The elderly gentleman, my grandfather, sits in a chair beside a gravestone. The grave belongs to his beloved wife.

His humsafar.

His gaze is distant. Perhaps he can see her beyond the horizon.

Perhaps he can see her right now.

◇◇◇

Sometimes, no matter what we do, a battle cannot be won. It is enough that we fought.

Sometimes, letting go is the victory.

Eventually we all reach the final threshold to the mystery we all will solve.

Others have jumped before us.

And we jump too.

My grandfather dies.

◇◇◇

Almost twenty years later now, I often see patients (and their families) who put up photos in their rooms.

I make it a point to always look at these photos. Sometimes I'll ask about them. Sometimes they make me smile. Sometimes they make me sad.

But I always look.

◇◇◇

I think that really seeing someone, as a person, is often the first step to helping and caring for them.

Photos can be a window.

They can show us who we were, who we are, and perhaps who we could be again.

The Bare-Knuckle Boxer

The first thing I notice about him is his oversize suit. Perhaps it fit him well once long ago, but it almost seems as if his frame shrank within it.

· He walks with a shuffling gait, his left arm slightly raised as if to ward off evil spirits.

I don't know him.

I'm at the grocery store, in line to pay. The man in the baggy suit stands behind me.

I don't know why, but I'm compelled to say something.

In retrospect, it was the suit. Something about it suggested a deep loneliness.

I open my mouth to speak, but he beats me to it.

◇◇◇

"How ya doin'?"

He has a gruff New Jersey accent. Unmistakable. It catches me off guard.

"I'm good. Ahh, find everything you needed?"

He nods. "Yep, yep. These prices though, they're killin' me these days."

I nod, and as I do so, I observe.

Every detail tells a story.

◇◇◇

His clothes are well-worn, the suit is rumpled and creased. It was expensive once, perhaps, long ago.

His shopping cart has canned pastas and junk-food meals. Low cost, low nutrition.

I also note a bag of meds from the pharmacy. Multiple prescriptions stapled together.

The line creeps forward. I look ahead at the person in front of me and then back at the man in the baggy suit.

He's elderly. If I had to guess, I'd say mid-70s, maybe more.

◇◇◇

He looks like he has something to say. He seems like he hasn't spoken to someone in a while.

"I used to box. Bare-knuckle." He grins, pretending to throw a jab or two at the air in front of him.

I wince. "Bare-knuckle? Sounds painful. Why not wear gloves?"

He scratches his jaw pensively. "I guess I figured if you're hurting someone, you should feel it too."

◇◇◇

I get home later that evening, unpacking my groceries, my mind still focused on the old man and his words.

I see him, with his oversize suit, his shopping cart with canned food and prescriptions.

His loneliness.

I keep thinking of him. Perhaps he reminds me of my father.

◇◇◇

The next day, at work, I'm playing the usual prior authorization game with an insurance company.

The phone tag followed by the peer-to-peer conversation with someone who isn't even in my field of medicine.

Before me on my desk sits a letter with "DENIAL" on it in bold print.

I'm finally taken off hold and connected to a human being. The specialist I'm supposed to peer-to-peer with.

They start asking me whether I've tried other treatments (I have) or multiple other drugs (I haven't tried EVERY possible alternative).

I see where this is going.

◇◇◇

My patient is in a lot of pain from a chronic inflammatory condition. The medication I'm trying to get would give them some relief.

I hear the baggy-suit man in my head: ". . . if you're hurting someone, you should feel it too."

I realize the insurance physician isn't feeling it.

◇◇◇

"Look," I say, "I know I haven't tried every alternative, and I know this drug is expensive, but my patient is in a lot of chronic pain and this could be huge for them. Imagine if it was your family member."

My plea for empathy sounds weak, even as it leaves my lips.

Silence.

"Okay, I'll approve it. Should be good to go in an hour or so."

And that's it.

Stunned, I thank them profusely. The call ends and I'm left with my thoughts.

How much pain could be averted if it didn't only fall on the most vulnerable among us?

If certain people felt it too.

◇◇◇

Before I said goodbye to the baggy-suit man at the grocery store, I asked him if I could help him load his groceries into his car.

"Thanks but no thanks." He waved me off, and I said goodbye.

The last I saw of him, he was counting out change from a faded brown wallet.

◇◇◇

I think often of the bare-knuckle boxer these days. I hope he's doing okay.

I think of what he said.

And every time I see all the ways in which our healthcare system is failing, every single day, I see who feels the pain.

Empathy isn't optional.

Change is coming.

It must.

Of Bluebirds and Bill

It's late fall, in the vast grasslands of the American West . . .

◇◇◇

A tiny turquoise-blue mountain bluebird lands on a branch. It's considered to be one of the most beautiful birds of the land.

The photographer holds her breath. She is motionless even though she knows the bird can't see her from so far away.

She brings it into focus and . . .

◇◇◇

I'm sitting in a special room. It's just outside the intensive care unit, adjacent to the waiting room.

Every ICU usually has one. Most ERs too.

The sign on the door says CONSULTATION ROOM, but that's only half the truth.

This is where lives are often changed forever.

◇◇◇

I have just had a conversation with a grieving family. The room is now empty except for me and the palliative care physician.

Well, I say it's empty, but grief leaves behind a palpable weight. A lingering reminder of the gravity of broken hearts.

Echoes of dreams undone.

◇◇◇

The palliative care doc is named Bill. He is a gifted clinician and thrives in his difficult role. He is somewhat baby-faced, appearing years younger than he really is.

His smile is warm and natural. He exudes empathy.

When he nods in understanding, you believe him.

◇◇◇

The two of us sit in silence for a few moments, in the consultation room.

My gaze is drawn to the pictures on the walls. Someone must like birds. One wall is covered in framed photos of them.

Brilliantly colored, they seem ready to take flight.

I envy their freedom.

◇◇◇

"One down, five to go." Bill breaks the silence with a sigh.

My eyebrows go up. "You have FIVE more family meetings today?"

He nods, taking off his glasses and rubbing his eyes. It's one of the few times I've seen him look weary.

"How do you do it, Bill?" I want to know.

◇◇◇

He smiles, and just like that his moment of vulnerability has passed.

"Well, Sayed, it's like any other difficult task, I suppose. I studied, I practiced, and I've had a *lot* of these conversations. I have a system now, an approach that seems to work pretty well."

He shrugs.

Listening, I nod, and then I probe a little more. "Does it wear on you? How do you do this without hurting?"

He is about to answer when he pauses for a moment.

Abruptly, he changes the subject. "You see those birds on the wall? Which one's your favorite?"

I look up.

◇◇◇

My favorite color has always been blue. One of the birds is a beautiful turquoise blue. It seems to be looking right at the camera, wings about to unfurl so it can take to the sky.

I point at it. "That one."

Bill squints at the frame. "Mountain bluebird. Nice."

◇◇◇

A thought occurs to me.

How many people have sat in this room and looked up at those bird photos while devastatingly powerful feelings cascade through them?

How many people have had a detached part of their mind focus on the bright colors to numb the pain?

Bill seems to sense my wandering mind.

He turns to me as he opens the door to leave the room.

"You asked me how I do this without hurting. The secret isn't in feeling nothing. It's just accepting what you feel. It can hurt, sometimes worse than others. And I accept it, whatever it is. I accept it."

He smiles.

◇◇◇

I smile in return, getting to my feet and following him out the door. I feel a strange warmth course through me, snaking down my spine and flooding outward.

As if I've learned some cosmic truth.

"Accept it."

I take one last look back at the photos on the wall, then leave.

◇◇◇

The mountain bluebird puffs up its chest as a cool breeze ruffles its feathers.

The photographer watches it through her lens and smiles as she snaps her photo.

Beautiful.

Suddenly the bluebird takes to the sky, flying off as if startled by the burden of all the grief it will never know.

Reset

The day I quit medicine was a Thursday, in 2004.

I was a freshly minted intern, arriving at my teaching hospital with that uniquely confusing mix of optimism and imposter syndrome that had defined my medical education.

I thought I was ready.

Instead, I was hopelessly lost.

As I sat on the Orange Line subway in Boston a thought occurred to me.

I could quit.

<><><>

Oh, how easy it could be. To just sit there and let the train doors close. Miss my stop.

A life without being paged or being on call. Without so many decisions carrying such grave consequences. With free weekends, always.

A life outside of medicine.

An actual life.

<><><>

And so I quit medicine.

Except not medicine on the whole.

Just medicine as I knew it.

I'd come too far, worked too hard, and cared too much to throw it all away now.

◇◇◇

I think about that moment often. How liberated I felt afterward.

I had searched so long for the heart of medicine, only to realize it was still beating within me.

My passion.

I decided to set myself free from the judgment of others.

I was here to learn, and I would.

◇◇◇

I got off the train, and went to work that day, and put all thoughts of quitting out of my mind.

Seventeen years later, I'm thinking about that moment again.

The reset.

I'm sitting in my car in the hospital parking lot and I don't want to get out. I want to keep driving.

◇◇◇

Something inside me isn't clicking the way it used to.

My job has become something it never was before and yet always was: just a job.

I don't know if it's the creeping cynicism. The looming specter of the Monster emerging from the shadows yet again.

The futility of it.

◇◇◇

Maybe it's knowing that I'm just a cog in the machine.

The constant noise, the climbing workload, the relentless pressure of bureaucracy and benchmarks.

I get out of my car, adjust my stethoscope around my neck, and head into the hospital.

Enough.

Time to find my faith.

◇◇◇

The funny thing about searching for something is that when you finally stop searching, that's when you see clearly. That's when you find it.

I get on the elevator and go up to one of the general medical floors.

I'm here to see a patient I've known for many years.

◇◇◇

She greets me with a smile, clasping my hand in both of hers.

Her room is filled with balloons that say "Happy Birthday!"

I glance at her date of birth on my sign-out list. It isn't her birthday.

55

"Who are the balloons for?"

She grins. "For Horatio!"

"Who's Horatio?"

◇◇◇

She smiles gleefully, like she's about to spill the beans on a major secret. "Horatio . . . is my kidney."

She's a kidney transplant recipient. I took care of her before her transplant and now after.

"You named your kidney?"

She nods.

I can't help but smile. "Why Horatio?"

◇◇◇

"I love *CSI* and my favorite character is Horatio."

As she speaks, a part of me is listening attentively. And a part of me is looking at these balloons that she got to celebrate the date of her kidney transplant.

Our worlds are built piece by piece, and every piece matters.

◇◇◇

We talk about her transplant function; she's doing better. Then I mention that she looks tired, and the conversation takes an unexpected turn.

"Of course I'm tired, Dr. T, I'm in a hospital."

I sigh. "No sleep?"

She scoffs. "In here? Forget it!"

We both fall silent.

◇◇◇

She breaks the silence. "You know, if hospitals really wanted to help patients, they'd let them sleep. Everyone else's schedule would just have to accommodate the patient's sleep."

I nod.

She continues. "And hospital food should be delicious! Not tasteless, but real!"

◇◇◇

I remain silent; she's on a roll.

"And you should encourage visitors. And make it easy to get your entire records for the stay. And have the most comfortable beds."

I finally speak up. "Good sleep, good eats, good sheets."

She laughs. "Yes! Just that. Simple things."

◇◇◇

I think about that. A hospital built from the ground up to center around the patients.

Entire medications, and labs, and rounding schedules, and the very architecture itself, built around the patient experience alone.

Gourmet food from a variety of cuisines.

Quality sheets.

◇◇◇

No crushing bills awaiting the patient on discharge. Fully covered care for everyone, without the psychological weight of how to pay.

Diverse and empathic staff not under the pressure of productivity/ profitability.

A reset on the modern hospital healthcare delivery system.

◇◇◇

We finish our visit, and I move on with my day.

The interaction with my patient has reminded me of something crucial.

So much power lies in our ability to reset.

Reset our minds. Reset our paradigms. Reset our systems.

Be the reset.

PART III

The Practice and the Passion

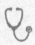

My earliest memories of medicine were always those of a destination I wanted to reach, a life goal. A distant mountaintop, wreathed in clouds and impossibly far away. As a child, then a young man, and even through medical school and residency and fellowship, medicine was always about The Next Step. It was always a goal to be attained, a light at the end of a tunnel that had consumed most of my lifetime.

And yet now, as I sit down and reflect on my writings about medicine, the moments that have come to linger in my mind, they're not linear at all. Instead of peering into a dark tunnel and seeing a light at the other end, I bring my eye to an opening and find myself looking into a kaleidoscope. This is how my mind sees medicine now: as a kaleidoscope of shifting moments, each catching the light in turn, uniquely beautiful, and forever changing. Moments upon moments, all existing at once, all connected.

In the introduction to the last part, I wrote about the sensation that I was losing a part of myself in the process of becoming a physician. While true on many levels, it doesn't mean that medicine never gave me anything back. The practice of medicine—and I practice it still—has been among the most immensely rewarding and enriching privileges of my life. It has taught me in so many ways and made me grow as a human being. Medicine can be a stern instructor, terrifying and unforgiving. But it can also be kind, and compassionate, and gentle in unexpected and crucial ways. Every day I learn more, and every day I am humbled by the limits of my knowledge. Medicine demands much, but it also allows for a depth and breadth of human experience that is unparalleled.

I began writing in medical school, to preserve my sense of self. I kept writing after I graduated, to preserve the sense of wonder that medicine was instilling within me. This process of preserving your passion is often preached as the antidote to burnout. They call it "remembering your why." Why you went into medicine in the first place. Why you chose this profession. Why you once valued it. Why you value it still.

These Vital Signs

It's a strange feeling to realize that everything you ever wanted and worked for was a dead end.

◇◇◇

It's 2003. I am a third-year medical student and I have no idea what to do with myself.

I thought I wanted to be a trauma surgeon. Some friends convinced me that only a scalpel can make a meaningful difference to a patient. Trauma surgery seemed like the kind of high-intensity field I might thrive in.

Only one problem, now that I'm trying it: I can't stand it. My whole life I've worked for this and now my plans have dissolved into . . . nothing.

◇◇◇

My mentor is a trauma surgeon. He is a kind man, soft-spoken with a wry sense of humor. Kind of the opposite of how I imagined surgeons being. I respect him immensely.

We check in from time to time. I lie and tell him I love surgery.

He seems pleased.

The truth is I don't have the passion for surgery that will sustain a career, or the manual dexterity, or the mindset. So what do I do? My fellow students seem relatively certain of their career choices.

But I am lost.

Finally, I come clean. I tell my mentor that surgery isn't for me. I expect him to be crestfallen, but he surprises me by laughing.

Apparently, he sensed my heart wasn't in it all along and was wondering how long I would keep up the charade.

He has some advice for me.

He tells me to work backward: Figure out what I definitely *don't* want to do and then choose from whatever is left over. Hmm.

◇◇◇

Surgery? No. Ob/gyn? It's sort of surgical, so no. Psychiatry? No, I'm no good at it. Family medicine? Maybe. Internal medicine? Maybe.

Pediatrics? This is a tough one. I really love kids. But pediatrics involves sick children and scared parents. I'm not strong enough.

◇◇◇

So, family medicine and internal medicine it is. Family medicine includes pediatrics in its scope, as well as some ob/gyn overlap, and that concerns me, so that leaves just internal medicine.

Okay. I have a direction now.

◇◇◇

I shall pursue internal medicine. Next step: I've always wanted to be a specialist within a field. So which internal medicine subspecialty shall I choose?

Ever since kidney physiology courses during the first year of med school, I can't stand the complex nature of the kidneys. They're a black box that I can't wrap my brain around.

Oh, and there's math. And chemistry. And yuck. Just yuck. I can't do it. I hate nephrology.

◇◇◇

But like most things in life, it's our mentors and role models who influence us. The greatest clinician I will ever meet is a nephrologist. When I am first assigned to his service for a med student rotation, my heart sinks. Anything but nephrology!

◇◇◇

I don't know it yet, but it is the rotation that will change my life and put me firmly on the trajectory I still follow to this day. I'll call the nephrologist Dr. G.

◇◇◇

Dr. G has that rarest combination of gifts. The ability, and the patience, to explain something clearly. He is kind, humble, and sharp as a hawk. He misses nothing; his clinical skills are superb. I witness him make challenging diagnoses swiftly and unerringly. Dr. G is everything I want to be.

◇◇◇

At the end of the rotation, he has me see a consult all by myself. When I am done, I am to formulate my own plan and present it.

I finish the consult and apply the principles that Dr. G has been teaching me. It is like a Rubik's Cube I am decoding, working the different permutations until I realize what makes sense.

I, a lowly medical student, am able to figure it out to the satisfaction of clinicians I respect. It is the happiest I've been in years, and it still gives me a rush to think about.

◇◇◇

Dr. G deconstructed my paradigm and rebuilt it slowly and carefully. Very quickly I realized that my "understanding" of the kidneys has been based on memorization, with little grasp of concepts and principles. I had started to see the kidneys in their context—their role in the body and the many ways they accomplish it—with clear eyes.

◇◇◇

For so long I had stumbled around in the minutiae, without a firm grasp of concepts and principles. Now I see the big picture: homeostasis and the means of achieving it.

◇◇◇

There are few things in life as gratifying as finally understanding something that you thought was beyond your reach. When I start to see past the math and the chemistry, I begin to see the precision, the intricacy, the magic, the incredible beauty of it.

◇◇◇

Nephrology is a discipline of awe-inspiring vastness and humbling complexity, of icy precision, and yet with key questions still unanswered, where relationships with patients can last a lifetime.

I am hooked.

I decide that I will pursue a career in nephrology once I am done with my internal medicine training.

◇◇◇

I've now been practicing nephrology for more than a decade.

It has been every bit as fulfilling as I imagined it would be as a medical student all those years ago. I can't imagine doing anything else. It has engaged my mind and challenges me every day.

I practice in a wide variety of clinical environments, from the ICU to the office, and I see patients on the total spectrum of illness severity, from asymptomatic conditions through kidney failure, dialysis, and transplantation.

◇◇◇

As part of what I do, I teach medical students and student nurse practitioners almost every day.
I see myself in them so often.

The same uncertainty.

The same hopes and fears.

◇◇◇

I tell them something Dr. G told me many years ago: Medicine, like life itself, is an exercise in managing uncertainty. It's okay to be unsure. It's okay not to have all the answers. And it's okay to figure things out as you go. Cultivate resilience and patience.

◇◇◇

There are people, principles, and purpose that nourish our spirits and illuminate the path forward. That show us the signs we look for to find our way.

These vital signs.

The Bouquet

The medical student shadowing me looks over my clinic schedule. She sighs.

"Dr. T, your youngest patient today is 70. Don't you get tired of only seeing older patients?"

It's a valid question. Elderly patients in my clinic, in general, tend to have a greater burden of chronic illness, more medications, more complexity, than their younger counterparts.

But I look down at my patient list and smile.

I don't see what she sees . . .

◇◇◇

At first glance, you might find Carl a bit intimidating.

Gruff and with a jaw that stubbornly juts out, as if daring you to try him, he seems perpetually irritated.

But Carl runs a dance studio and still dances every day.

At 80.

And when he smiles, the sun shines for him.

◇◇◇

Gladys shows me a photograph.

She seems proud, and I regard it carefully. It's a black-and-white shot of a concert. A young singer has his back to the camera. The rest is a sea of screaming fans.

A young Gladys is in the front row, clearly visible.

The singer?

Elvis.

◇◇◇

John and Lucy always come to their appointments together.

Sitting beside each other, they hold hands. Every. Single. Appointment.

I'm always moved by how quiet each one is when it's the other one's "turn" during the appointment.

They've been married for sixty years.

◇◇◇

Anjali brings me food, without fail.

All sorts of delicious desserts that she cooks herself. I once tried to refuse (I'm trying to lose weight), but she looked like she would cry.

Her husband explains: Their son died in a car accident years ago. She used to cook for him.

◇◇◇

Howard can barely hear me.

Every single visit he apologizes for being almost deaf and explains, "I LOST MOST OF MY HEARING IN THE WAR!"

He has a photo in his wallet, of him in military uniform. I ask him how he won the medals he's wearing.

He grins.

"I KEPT MY HEAD DOWN!"

◇◇◇

Alma has an amazing knack for gardening.

I look forward to her appointments so that I can learn more about what's in season in south Texas this time of year.

We discuss how therapeutic it is to watch a plant sprout.

Her secret?

"Love."

Every living thing needs love to grow.

◇◇◇

Steve plays tennis almost every day.

He's in his late 70s, and one day, finally, I have to suggest that he start toning it down. I'm worried about dehydration.

He says he understands. He'll tone it down. He promises.
Then he starts walking his dogs for four miles a day.

◇◇◇

Mike is one of the kindest human beings I've ever met.
He brings my entire office staff a bouquet of red and white roses every single visit.
His smile is gentle, his eyes are kind.
He asks me how *I'm* doing at the start of every appointment and really wants to know.

◇◇◇

One day Mike doesn't show for his appointment.
I know something's wrong when his wife sends us a bouquet of red and white roses, and a note.
"Mike passed away in his sleep. It was peaceful. He loved you and your office staff very much. Thank you."
My heart is broken.

◇◇◇

"Don't you wanna see younger patients? Maybe simpler patients? At least sometimes?"
I look up from my patient list, and my reverie, to respond.
"This . . . is a privilege."
My student smiles, but the look in her eyes tells me she doesn't quite seem to understand.
I hope that someday she will.

Where Hearts Beat Strongly

He suffers from a rare cardiomyopathy and has been hospitalized for weeks.

He awaits a transplant.

His heart is failing.
He has been admitted for inotropic therapy, medications that help the heart pump more effectively.

He's 23.

◇◇◇

I am a resident at the heart failure service. It's known as the "rock garden" because of how chronically ill and complex the patients are.

The hospital is a miserable place to be in general.

Doubly so when you're young.

The Wi-Fi reception is lousy here, so his PlayStation is useless for online gaming.

◇◇◇

We forge an unlikely friendship, primarily because he loves video games and so do I.

After finishing rounds, I join him for two-player games, since the internet won't let him play against online players.

He has everything hooked up to the TV in his room.

We game hard.

◇◇◇

Competing against someone is an interesting means to get to know them.

In a strange way, rivals often have a more intimate understanding and appreciation of each other than friends do.

We compete against each other almost every day.

He usually wins. Easily.

◇◇◇

"Come on, Doc," he says, grinning, "I'm trying to make you better. Learn from me!"

"I don't think gaming is what I'm supposed to be learning from you" is my frustrated reply, as I lose yet again.

He seems genuinely happy when he wins, and I have to smile.

I want to help him, badly.

◇◇◇

As we game, we talk about everything.

He tells me about his dreams of going into advertising, specifically for Snickers. He has a killer idea for a jingle.

I didn't know "Snickers" could rhyme with so many words . . .

He pulls a dirty trick on me one day.

I'm actually winning the game for once, and he suddenly clutches his chest and yells, "Doc!"

All the color drains from my face as I whip around to face him. "What?! Are you okay?!"

He laughs, and defeats me easily.

I sigh, relieved.

A moment comes to pass one day when, for the first time, he becomes vulnerable in front of me.

I'm watching him play the game by himself, and he turns to look at me.

"Do you really think I'll ever get this transplant?"

He's a big guy, but in that moment, he seems so small.

It's easy for me to forget how young he is. And he's always so confident and cocky when he's gaming. His momentary vulnerability catches me off guard.

I do something I'll regret for the rest of my life.

I brush off his fear.

"Pfffst! Now win this game, it's so close!"

I can see him almost visibly flinch and then retreat into his shell. Just like that we are back to being gaming buddies.

But we were never just buddies, were we?

I am his doctor. He is my patient.

And he tried to talk to me about his genuine fears, and I brushed them aside.

◇◇◇

One morning I pick up my sign-out from the night float, and she seems sad.

"I'm sorry." Her eyes are bloodshot, tired.

Something about a code blue.

Something about a death.

I can't hear her. My heart is in my throat.

I make my way up to his room.

It's empty.

◇◇◇

This doesn't make any sense.

I was just laughing with him about Snickers rhyming with knickers. We just gamed together.

He was going to get transplanted.

He was doing so well.

This doesn't make any sense.

The empty room. The blank space on my census list. None of it.

◇◇◇

The rest of the day is a blur.

I am numb to everything. I can't summon any feelings except disbelief.

Nothing makes sense.

On the train ride home that night, I find myself resenting the other passengers and their healthy cardiac output.

How dare they take it for granted.

◇◇◇

When I get home, I collapse on my couch, not bothering to change out of my scrubs or take off my shoes.

I fall asleep like that, without moving.

My alarm wakes me up at 5:00 AM, and I steel myself to go back to the hospital and to the new patient in his room.

◇◇◇

I don't cry until many weeks later.

Something innocuous sets it off. A Snickers bar in a gas station, of all places. I buy every last one they have, bags full.

Then I sit in my car and grip the steering wheel until my knuckles turn white, and cry. And cry. And cry.

◇◇◇

"I'm trying to make you better. Learn from me!"

I know you were talking about a video game.

But I also know your words will never leave me.

I am so deeply sorry.

I hope someday I'll see you again, in a place where the Wi-Fi is always great and all hearts beat strongly.

A Dog Named Tesla

My last patient of the day sits across from me in the exam room. He's a hulking tree trunk of a man, his arms are folded across his massive chest, and he has his usual look of irritation. He leans back in his chair.

We begin the rituals of the office visit.

<><><>

I follow him for chronic kidney disease, but the story of our interactions could be encapsulated in one issue: smoking. He has been a remarkably motivated patient. He lost weight with diet and exercise. He gave up his heavy soda intake and now drinks mainly water.

But smoking is a bridge too far.

<><><>

Some patients get angry when we start discussing smoking cessation. They tell me that no matter what I say, they won't quit it. And they want me to *quit* talking about it.

Yet you always have to dig a little deeper.

<><><>

The man sitting before me is physically imposing, rippling with muscle. But he's a gentle giant. He's a biker, so he can ride with a group against child abuse. Through our many office visits and conversations, I discover that he didn't start smoking until his pet dog died. He lives alone now.

Our stories define us.

Taking away his smoking is taking away something more than just cigarettes. A coping mechanism. I ask him for the first time if we can just talk about his dog for a bit, and the floodgates open. The usually impassive face softens and he becomes almost childlike in his enthusiasm to show photos.

Then he shows me the photo taken of him cradling her the day she was taken to be euthanized. I look up at him and see his eyes filled with tears.

And suddenly I understand clearly. The quiet anger, the folded arms, the smoking, all of it.

We grieve in so many different ways.

◇◇◇

I don't talk to him about smoking anymore after that. Instead, every time I see him in the clinic, I let him talk, and I look at old photos of him and his dog, Lucy.
What intensely lonely lives some of us live.
So many of us.

◇◇◇

One day, during another follow-up visit, I suggest perhaps getting another dog. Not to replace Lucy—no one could ever replace her—but just to have another furry friend to provide nonjudgmental love.

At first his silence makes me think I've overstepped. But then he exhales, a long shuddering breath, and admits that he has thought about it.

At his next office visit six months later, I notice something immediately. He doesn't reek of cigarette smoke anymore.

◇◇◇

As I listen to his heart, I notice that the bulge in his shirt pocket isn't a pack of cigarettes; it's a box of Tic Tacs.

◇◇◇

We go over his kidney function, blood pressure, anemia, vitamin D, and make plans for his next follow-up.

◇◇◇

As he gets up to leave, he asks me a question. "Doc, why did you stop asking about the smoking?"

"Because I know you quit."

He grins. "Maybe I just washed my clothes real good."

Considering this, I sigh.

He laughs. "Just messin'."

◇◇◇

He shows me photos of his new canine buddy, named Tesla, because he can't afford the car but now he can still say he owns a Tesla and impress the ladies.

I groan, but can't help but laugh at his newfound cheesy sense of humor.

"Cigarettes were getting too expensive anyway, I just bought a Tesla . . ."

Unexpected Storms, Toy Boats, Safe Harbors

It starts with a subtle unease.

She can't describe what's wrong with her because she isn't even sure there's anything wrong.

Something just feels . . . "off."

Maybe she's a little tired. Maybe she's a little stressed. Maybe her college classes are too much.

Who knows?

◇◇◇

As the weeks pass, the vague unease coalesces into a sinking fear.

Something is definitely wrong.

She's tired, all the time. Her appetite is gone. She withdraws from her social life, and her grades start to dip.

Deep inside her, an illness is beginning to take hold . . .

◇◇◇

She goes to see her primary care doctor. Tests are run and everything is normal. By now she has a cough and sinusitis. She is started on antibiotics.

Despite the antibiotics she feels worse.

She has low-grade fevers. Her joints ache. Her cough won't go away.

◇◇◇

She goes back to her doctor. More tests are run.

Her platelet count is a little high, but things don't look too bad. Then a marker for inflammation is checked (an ESR), and it is very high.

She is started on empiric steroids and is referred to see rheumatology.

◇◇◇

For a while, she feels great. The steroids make everything better.

She starts eating again. She is able to go to class. Her fevers subside.

But the improvement is short-lived.

Her cough comes back with a vengeance. She goes to the ER and is diagnosed with pneumonia.

◇◇◇

She is discharged with another course of antibiotics. She takes these dutifully, but she has a feeling they're doing nothing.

Days pass.

She notices a rash.

Her urine is looking red, almost rusty.

Deep inside her, the illness is progressing rapidly now . . .

◇◇◇

She's scared. She knows something is deeply wrong. She calls her primary care doctor, who tells her to come in tomorrow to be seen or go to the ER.

In tears, she calls her mother.

She's short of breath on the phone.

As she hangs up, she starts coughing.

Her sputum is bloody.

◇◇◇

The human body has a remarkable ability to hold the line, to compensate.
There are backup systems, and backups to the backups.

But once the tipping point is reached, things can fall apart devastatingly fast.

I am asleep when my phone rings.

◇◇◇

When I see her for the first time, she is already on a ventilator. Her family is at the bedside.

Inside her body, an avalanche of organ dysfunction is taking place, stemming from an immune system run amok.

Blood vessels are under attack. She is bleeding internally.

Untreated, she will die, soon.

The working diagnosis is a pulmonary-renal syndrome, a vasculitis, a disease of the immune system.

Together with the pulmonary/critical care team, we begin treatment.

Dialysis. Plasma exchange. Steroids. Immunosuppressive therapy.

◇◇◇

There is a stillness that comes over a room where the greatest battles of life and death are being fought.

We all sense it instinctively, the weight of it.

It is a battle that has been fought since the dawn of time.

The only sounds are monitor beeps and ventilator hisses.

She lies motionless, tethered to the machines.

There are only the faintest signs of life. The rise and fall of her chest. The delicate flutter of the jugular venous pulsation.

The tracings on the monitor that remind us that a heart still beats, that signs are still vital.

◇◇◇

I get to know her better in the days that follow, through her family.

Her room is covered in photographs, and I look into each one. Her mother explains them, often laughing, sometimes crying.

They tell the story of a life filled with a gentle love and a burning purpose.

◇◇◇

One photo in particular sticks out to me.

A photo of her, as a young girl. She is kneeling beside a pond, reaching out to a toy boat.

It's raining. The little toy boat is being battered by the raindrops.

She offers it shelter from the storm and holds out her hands.

◇◇◇

The worst of her storm passes, in time, as her immune system is finally held in check and pulled back onto the rails.

She wakes up, as her sedation is weaned. She smiles at her family, as their tears stream down.

She offers a thumbs-up.

She is a fighter, and I am awed.

◇◇◇

Eventually she is successfully extubated. Her kidneys start working again, and we stop dialysis. She is transferred out of the ICU.

She asks me what happened to her, why did she get so sick.

As I try to explain, I see a clarity in her eyes, a wonder at her own unraveling.

◇◇◇

A year later, and the young woman I see in the clinic looks nothing like the weakened patient who was in the hospital for so long and needed weeks of physical therapy.

She is doing well in college.

She is upbeat and happy.

◇◇◇

Her father accompanies her to every clinic visit. He rarely says anything, just smiles and listens and thanks me at the end.

Today, however, he has something to say. He waits until his daughter has left the room, then turns to me.

"Dr. T, what were her odds?"

◇◇◇

"Her odds?" I quirk a brow.

"What were the chances that she could have died from this?"

"Ahh . . . it varies. She's young. She's a fighter . . ." I trail off.

He looks at me and nods, an understanding passing between us.

Trivia Like Flowers

There are always questions at the end of the visit.

It's only natural. Nobody remembers everything. I'm used to clarifying and reiterating.

But your question catches me off guard.

"Did you know that hummingbirds remember every single flower they've ever visited?"

◇◇◇

I smile, then shake my head. "No, I didn't know that."

You nod at me. "Well, it's true. I'm gonna send you a bill now."

I laugh, and the layered masks muffle the sound.

I was consulted because your kidney function is dropping.

Clear yellow urine now turning dark amber.

◇◇◇

Your room is on a COVID unit.

The plastic sheets you have to zipper yourself through. The cool hiss of the air flow. Donning and doffing.

There was a time when this was a pulse-quickening ritual, when adrenaline would flow.

Now it is a necessary nuisance.

Numbing.

◇◇◇

Every time I see you, the visit finishes with an exchange of trivia.

You tell me something I didn't know.

I try to tell you something equally interesting.

It's a sort of game. A challenge.

I realize that it's something I'm looking forward to every day.

A little joy.

◇◇◇

Late in the evening, when I get home, I sit down with some books and skim through for interesting tidbits I could use.

Schott's Original Miscellany is a godsend, as is *Guinness World Records*.

I enjoy the peace.

No screens. No one monetizing my attention.

Just pages turning.

◇◇◇

"Did you know Bluetooth is named for a Viking king, and the symbol is his initials in runic form?"

"Did you know that a group of ferrets is called a 'business'?"

"Did you know in Japan they have cube-shaped watermelons?"

"Did you know that M&M's stands for 'Mars' & 'Murrie'?"

◇◇◇

Every time I see you, I'm well prepared with a piece of trivia, and you always have some obscure fact ready.

I never ask you where this pastime of yours started. I just go with it.

It makes you smile.

And it makes me smile too.

At least for as long as life lets us.

◇◇◇

The last time I see you is a Friday. You're more tired than I remember you being.

I don't remember the piece of trivia I share with you. Perhaps something about Scotland.

For the first time, you don't have any trivia for me.

You just thank me for taking care of you.

◇◇◇

I never see you again.

When I come back to work after my weekend off, your name isn't on the list.

This happens with numbing regularity in the age of COVID.

Still, I hope.

I hope you got better, that you were discharged home.

That you're enjoying trivia with your family.

◇◇◇

But when I look you up, I see the dreaded pop-up window on my computer that sounds unreasonably cheerful in my head.

"This patient is deceased!"

And I just sit and feel the color drain from my vision slowly.

Did you know, over a million people have died from COVID-19 in America?

Do you know?

◠◠◡◠

As death lingers in the hallways and steps into the rooms, I think of you.

I remember you and your trivia questions like flowers.

Like a hummingbird, I remember every single one.

What Did It Take?

"They just told me I have cancer. It's everywhere in my body. And you say you're a kidney doctor? What the hell are you doing here?"

His voice is gruff, and as he looks at me, I feel the weight of his gaze.

For a moment I hesitate, then ask.

"Mind if I sit down?"

◇◇◇

"What do I care, you're gonna be gone in ten seconds anyways. Nobody sticks around, tell that chickenshit doctor who hasn't seen me in three days that I know he's gonna bill me anyways."

I don't speak. Not now.

He continues. "Sit down, tell me how bad my kidneys are."

◇◇◇

The harsh truth is that my day would be easier if I didn't sit down.

If I just stood at his bedside and spoke fast, did a perfunctory physical exam, and moved on.

The system incentivizes me to see more people, faster. And the faster I'm done, the faster I can go home.

◇◇◇

Some days, yeah, all I want to do is go home early.

Some days.

I sit down and make eye contact. His gaze is angry, accusing, and beneath it all, afraid.

He is twice my age, and for a moment, I see myself through his eyes.

Young. Detached.

An agent of the system.

◇◇◇

I start talking, and almost immediately I'm interrupted. I knew he was angry, but I underestimated his rage.

This isn't just about the cancer. I understand.

There's grief here too. An undercurrent of grief, far more than I can know.

My instinct is to deflect.

◇◇◇

I want to tell him this isn't my fault and to quickly launch into one of my pre-canned speeches about kidney function and lab values.

To face emotion like his, head-on, can be terrifying.

Instead, a distant memory calms me.

My father's voice: "What did it take?"

91

When I was a child, I was at a party at a friend's house. There was a toy my mom had bought for me before the party. A ninja turtle, the purple one, Donatello.

At the party we watched *Teenage Mutant Ninja Turtles.*

And my friend said his favorite turtle was Donatello.

◇◇◇

As we were leaving the party, my friend saw the toy in my car and asked if he could borrow it.

His parents were pretty strict when it came to expenditures on toys. I knew he didn't have any ninja turtles.

Impulsively, I gave him Donatello.

On the drive home my dad smiled.

◇◇◇

"Did you see how happy you made that kid? You make someone happy like that, and it's special. And what did it take? Just a toy."

I nod.

"What did it take?" becomes a mantra for me.

How simple kindness can be, how easy, if you're mindful.

How positivity can ripple.

◇◇◇

My patient's gaze is no longer angry, or scared, but defiant. "So . . . what do you have to say about my kidneys?"

I tell him I'm sorry. That I hear him. And that actually his kidneys are doing pretty well.

He laughs sardonically. "Well, at least I got that going for me . . ."

◇◇◇

As the days pass, I go in and see my gruff patient in the hospital every day.

I know visits with him will take longer than those with any other patient on my list, primarily because I am one of the only docs he gets to see.

His other docs tend to round when he's asleep or sedated.

◇◇◇

We start having conversations that extend beyond the scope of his illness.

Conversations about life and our experiences.

We have unexpected things in common, and discovering them is a unique joy.

The day finally comes when I take a seat in his room for the last time.

◇◇◇

He has chosen to pursue hospice care and will be going home to his family.

I am grateful that he will be at peace, surrounded by people who love him.

He thanks me for spending time with him and "facing the music" as he gruffly puts it.

I thank him for his kindness.

◇◇◇

All I did was sit down in his room every day. Sit down and listen, and eventually talk.

There was no great medicine I prescribed, no cure.

And yet I faced the music with him, and it was my privilege.

As I get up to leave, we say our goodbyes. I feel a wave of grief.

◇◇◇

Days later, as I round in the hospital, I find myself glancing at his room number when I walk past it.

Remembering.

The longer you practice medicine, the more faces never leave you. The more memories linger.

"What did it take?"

Nothing at all.

Time.

Every last thing.

A Casual Cruelty

Why do we do the things we do?

What do we really believe in?

My next clinic patient is one I've known for many years. He is visiting me today via Zoom.

I always look forward to talking to him.

◇◇◇

As soon as the visit begins, I notice that his camera is angled off-center so I can't get a clear look at his face.

I ask if he can adjust it, but he says he's having technical issues.

No problem. I can adapt.

It isn't just the camera though.

Something feels off today.

◇◇◇

Almost immediately I can tell that he sounds subdued. He isn't cracking his usual jokes.

I'm comfortable with silence, even in the heart of a busy clinic day.

Silence is often where the healing happens.

After asking how he's doing, I let the silence between us grow.

The question, when he asks it, is one I don't expect.

"Doc, which kills you faster? Blood pressure you don't control or blood sugar you don't control?"

The surprise on my face must register, because he explains further.

"I just can't afford all these medications anymore."

◇◇◇

He continues.

"The way I see it, Doc, I only need to stick around 4 or 5 more years. That's how long my pet dog has left, then I ain't got no more family and it's me all on my own. So I figure maybe take the diabetes ones and skip the blood pressure? Or every other day?"

◇◇◇

As I review his meds and start discussing our options with him, he adds one last remark.

"And I'm real sorry, Doc. I know we go back a ways, but I can't afford my co-pay. I'll pay you later. Promise."

And just like that, I understand why his camera is angled.

◇◇◇

And just like that, I'm again struck by the cruel illusion of what I do.

The system I'm part of.

This patient did everything right: got insurance, paid his taxes. And he still has to barter years of his life.

And he can't bring himself to look me in the eyes as he does so.

◇◇◇

Our healthcare system is too often unethical, immoral, unsustainable.

The insurance paradigm is focused on revenue generation. It strips the basic human dignity from patients to the point where they can't even make eye contact anymore.

I know that I'm part of this system.

◇◇◇

He's old enough to be my father. Some part of me imagines that he is my father. Tears threaten my vision as a hot anger floods me.

Now I wish I could angle my camera away.

I ask him if I can write about him. Because people need to know.

His response lingers with me.

◇◇◇

"Sure you can, Doc. But people already know. Lots of people deal with this. It ain't that people don't know. It's just that nobody cares. Nobody gives enough of a damn to change anything. Nobody . . . cares."

The visit ends.

My Zoom window closes.

His window closes too.

◇◇◇

I feel it.

There's something insidious here.

A casual cruelty we're all complicit in.

"I can't go to rehab, insurance won't cover it."

"Insurance won't pay for that medication."

"I can't afford any of this."

"I'm uninsured."

This isn't right. None of this is right.

Our lives mean more than this. Our systems must change.

PART IV

The Pandemic and the Precipice

In late 2019 the first reports of a novel coronavirus emerged out of Wuhan, China. In the days and weeks and months that followed, it became increasingly clear that this new pathogen had the potential to wreak havoc on a global scale that hadn't been seen in more than a century.

Like most Americans, I followed the news closely as COVID-19 began burning its way through the world. I'm not really one for premonitions, but I distinctly remember a sickening, sinking feeling as I watched grainy footage of Chinese military vehicles moving through a locked-down Wuhan. The sense of things spiraling, unraveling, rapidly. As if the ground was shifting beneath me almost imperceptibly. Talking my fears over with a friend one night, I blurted out a number. "I think a million Americans could die from this." His response was silence. I wasn't sure in that moment if I was being an alarmist.

As the first patients began to be admitted with the COVID+ diagnoses, and our ICUs began to fill up, my writing output increased exponentially. The truth was that I'd never been through an experience like this before. None of us had. My writing on Twitter became urgent, a documentation of the raging inferno we found ourselves in. But I also wrote for other reasons.

Writing became more than a hobby or pastime for me during this period—it was a lifeline. I came home exhausted every day, unable to process anything beyond what I wanted to eat for dinner (and sometimes not even that). As I lay down in bed and stared up at the ceiling, my mind would begin to unpack the day's events and invariably I would get the urge to write. The words would pour out of me as I raged, grieved, and remembered. They were my therapy. Without my writing, I would have been lost.

In March of 2021, the toll of COVID-19 became devastatingly personal for me. My uncle, a soft-spoken and kind man, died of the disease. His death was just another data point, another name and number added to a mortality total in some ledger somewhere, but it was also a gaping hole in my heart. My sleep, already erratic, became nonexistent. As my family grieved his death, I started shutting down, emotionally, psychologically, spiritually. Any fear I had of COVID itself was being replaced with a hard and bitter anger, and eventually numbness.

If it felt like I had lost a part of myself during my medical education, that feeling was vastly more intense during the worst waves of the COVID-19 pandemic and with the death of my beloved uncle. In one of my writings, I mused that I was regressing and devolving from a human being into a combination of scar tissue and raw nerves, numb to the world yet still coursing with pain. Empathy, which had been a significant portion of the why of medicine for me, was now crushing me. Through necessity I began to grow emotionally detached and distant from my work. But my writing didn't.

At the time of this writing, COVID-19 is still killing hundreds if not thousands of people every day. My fervent prayer is that someday this pandemic will be far in the past and we will have learned the valuable and difficult lessons it had to teach us.

I hope that someday my COVID-19 stories are nothing more than memories left to bear witness.

The Monster

I turn off the lights.

These bulbs are old, not the newer LEDs. There is a lingering glow as the hot tungsten filaments gradually cool.

I watch them as the room slowly goes dark.

A lingering glow . . . and then nothing.

I am exhausted, but I can't sleep.

A monster awaits.

◇◇◇

Morning comes far sooner than it has any right to, and before I know it I'm back in the hospital.

It's almost like my time away from this place was the dream and the hospital is my waking reality.

N95 on, surgical mask over it.

Face shield for when it's time.

Armor up.

◇◇◇

You don't face the monster without armor. Even if it's in short supply, you reuse what you have, and you find a way to make it work.

And you don't face the monster alone.

The intensivist sits with me in the dictation room.

She is a seasoned veteran.

She leads naturally.

◇◇◇

I've known her for five years now. She is kind, with a smile that brightens the room. Like when she shows me photos of her son's graduation or a funny meme.

But beneath the kind smile is a steely resolve.

And above the mask her green eyes are twin pools of calm strength.

◇◇◇

Something is different today.

Something in the air, quite literally.

The monster is on the prowl.

The intensivist is more stressed than I can remember her being. Her smile is thin.

"Tubed several so far. Floor people decompensating. ER is packed."

Short, staccato updates.

◇◇◇

We are in the dictation room together. A sort of fishbowl in the middle of the ICU, with large glass windows.

A nurse comes up and opens the door, her voice terse. "Doc, we need you out here."

"Coming." She gets up quickly, grabbing her stethoscope.

I follow, to see.

◇◇◇

The COVID rooms are sealed, negative pressure rooms, constantly keeping air flowing inward.

Outside the doors are sets of IV pumps, so they can be adjusted without going inside.

Face shields hang on makeshift hooks when not in use, names written on them with a Sharpie.

◇◇◇

One of the patients is not yet intubated, but is experiencing that rapid decline that is the hallmark of the monster attacking aggressively.

The breathing is becoming shallow, labored, despite multiple interventions.

The ICU team prepares for another intubation

Armor up.

◇◇◇

I am a nephrologist by training, but I am also board certified in internal medicine, and I spend a fair amount of my time practicing critical care medicine.

I sit down at the table outside the room. Backup, just in case things go sideways.

The team preps rapidly, smoothly.

◇◇◇

To enter the monster's lair and perform an "aerosolizing procedure" requires special precautions.

The team (the doc, a respiratory therapist, and an ICU nurse) wears PAPR hoods.

PAPR—Powered Air-Purifying Respirator—running on batteries.

They put them on in silence.

◇◇◇

Once the PAPR is active you can't hear much while wearing it. The whirring of the fan drowns out a lot of sound.

To make sure they can hear one another, the team dials in to a special number and tapes their headphones to their ears so they won't dislodge accidentally.

◇◇◇

Sitting outside the room, I dial in to the line on my phone, and I can hear them too.

They enter the room, the door sliding open slightly with a hiss.

Now they are in the monster's lair.

"You got everything?"
"Yup."
"I'm going to move fast."
"Ready to position."
"On it."

◇◇◇

They talk to one another with the calm efficiency of a cohesive team of professionals, at the peak of their expertise.

I can hear the patient through their mics. She's gasping with each labored breath.

"Ohgodohgodohgodohgodohgod—"

Her voice is growing quieter.

Ominous.

◇◇◇

Sometimes when people sound quieter and calmer during a respiratory issue it's a sign of impending doom.

You can't make noise if you can't breathe.

The team moves rapidly.

"Etomidate."
"Yes."
"Succs."
"In."

The intensivist's eyes are keenly focused as she intubates.

She is a mother, and just a few weeks ago she was proudly showing me her son's socially distanced graduation photos.

As I watch her team save a life, I wonder how I could make people see.

The risks that some have to take because of the simple steps that others wouldn't.

◇◇◇

Afterward we are back sitting in the dictation room. She reviews the chest X-ray to confirm the placement of the breathing tube.

"Looks good."

She exhales deeply, rubbing her eyes. Then she looks up.

"You okay, Sayed? Did you eat something?"

Her empathy is her strength.

◇◇◇

Before either of us can grab a bite to eat, another emergency page.

Another patient beginning to succumb.

The monster is raging like a wildfire.

She opens a small package of gummy bears and pops a handful in her mouth.

The sugar will help.

Time to go.

Armor up.

◇◇◇

The day passes in this way and turns to night.

Not every life has been saved. People have died today.

My fatigue is the kind that makes my soul feel shallower.

I am hollow.

The work isn't done, but it isn't ours anymore. Backup arrives in the form of the on-call team.

◇◇◇

Before we leave for the day, I tell the intensivist I'm going to write about her.

She is exhausted, her face marked with the indentations of her PPE, but she smiles.

"Aw, really? Be sure to tell your readers to wear their masks."

I nod. "You got it."

Time to go home.

◇◇◇

In the elevator to the garage, I run into the patient's respiratory therapist.

I tell her I'm going to write about the day.

I ask her if she has any messages.

She nods, and her smile is faint.

"Wear your fucking masks. Distance. None of this had to happen. None of it."

◇◇◇

As I drive home I pass a restaurant less than a few blocks from the hospital.

It's packed, and I can see only a few masks as I drive by.

The thought occurs to me.

The monster isn't just in those hospital rooms.

Everywhere, people are risking other people's lives.

◇◇◇

I finally get home.

Get ready for bed.

I turn off the lights.

These bulbs are old, not the newer LEDs. There is a lingering glow as the hot tungsten filaments gradually cool.

I watch them as the room slowly goes dark.

A lingering glow . . . and then nothing.

A monster awaits.

These Crooked Paths

The phone call comes in the early morning hours.

It is a call they've been dreading.

His wife's hands shake as she fumbles with her phone, trying to use FaceTime, her vision blurry with tears.

He sits silently beside her.

While she sobs, he remembers.

These crooked paths.

◇◇◇

He is fed up with COVID.

There's only so much a man can take. Everything seems uncertain, and everything seems unfair.

Every decision to reopen and then roll back hits him in his gut. This sense that nobody knows what they're doing.

Enough.

He's going out.

◇◇◇

His wife asks him where he's going.

"Just a drive. I gotta get outta here for a bit."

She asks him to wear his mask, and he says something gruffly under his breath as he leaves.

His car comes to life with a roar, and he accelerates out of the driveway and into the night.

◇◇◇

The open road is comforting.

He lowers his windows and turns up the music. Life is a highway.

The wind ruffles his hair.

Freedom.

He smiles and breathes in deeply. No quarantine here. No masks. No contradictions.

On a whim, he decides to stop at a diner.

◇◇◇

He's trying to lose weight, eat healthier. His wife is big on a meal-planning kick. Everything is steamed.

Well, tonight, he's in the mood for a milkshake and some fries, and that's what he's going to get.

He parks his car and gets out.

He leaves his mask.

◇◇◇

It's not that he has anything against the masks themselves. Heck, he honestly doesn't even notice it after wearing it a while.

But it's what the mask symbolizes to him now. This unending saga that's cost him his job, his freedom.

Besides, nobody at this diner is masked up.

◇◇◇

He steps inside and his smile broadens. The diner is packed. It feels so good to be part of a crowd.

As if the pressing together of humanity is one giant rebuke to this moment, this monster.

He sits down and orders his food.

It arrives, and it is delicious.

◇◇◇

He pays the bill, nods a smile of thanks to the server, and gets up to go.

The moment that will change his life forever happens so innocuously that he doesn't even realize it at first.

In the years ahead, this is the moment he will revisit repeatedly.

Someone nearby coughs.

◇◇◇

He gets home and feels a twinge of guilt as he realizes his wife left food out for him and has already gone to sleep.

His mom, however, is still awake and watching TV in the living room.

She's been living with them since his dad died last year.

"Good night, Mom."

"G'night."

◇◇◇

His dreams are troubled that night. He has been having vivid nightmares lately, but this one is just strange.

He's lost in the woods. Darkness and shadows surround him.

The path ahead should be clear, but it isn't. It's crooked and leads him in circles.

He can't sleep.

◇◇◇

A week later, he wakes up one morning feeling immensely fatigued and achy.

His wife has already gone to work. She is an essential worker. Doubly essential now that he's been laid off.

He groans and sits up, rubbing his temples.

He can hear his mom in the kitchen.

◇◇◇

As he finishes brushing his teeth, he feels his muscles aching badly all over.

A chill runs through him.

A gnawing realization.

"Mom?"

She calls back from the kitchen, "Yes?"

"Do you have Dad's old thermometer?"

"Yes. Why?"

"Nothing, just wanna check something."

◇◇◇

It's an old mercury thermometer. He rinses it off, then puts it under his tongue.

His mom has already felt his forehead with the back of her hand and says he feels fine to her.

As he waits, she starts telling one of her rambling stories.

For once, he listens.

◇◇◇

"You know, when you were a little boy, your dad and I almost lost you. We had taken you to the park and looked away for just a moment and . . . poof! You vanished into the woods! There were all these crooked paths going in circles. Thank God we found you."

She smiles.

He would have smiled too, except that he stopped listening toward the end of the story. Because he's staring at the mercury in the thermometer.

100.9.

No way.

He looks at his mom. Her frail frame, her wispy white hair, the way her back bows into thin shoulders.

Oh, no.

◇◇◇

There are some nightmares you can't wake up from.

There are some moments in your life that get burned into your psyche with such terrible clarity.

When he's diagnosed with COVID-19, it barely registers in his brain.

It's his mom testing positive later that crushes him.

◇◇◇

His wife is convinced it was neighbors who walked too close by, damn them.

She asks him about his mask, and he lies and says he's always worn it.

He doesn't tell her about the diner. He can't.

His mom is hospitalized a week later.

He can't visit her. Nobody can.

◇◇◇

The phone call comes in the early morning hours.

It is a call they've been dreading.

His wife's hands shake as she fumbles with her phone, trying to use FaceTime, her vision blurry with tears.

He sits silently beside her.

While she sobs, he remembers.

Those crooked paths.

The Meaning of Loss

It starts raining as I'm driving home from the hospital.

Normally the rain is background noise.

Today it's different. The raindrops are splattering against the windshield with an urgency, an intensity.

As if they have something to say.

I listen.

<><><>

My mind focuses. The steady beat of the rain reminding me of something.

Raindrops. Tears.

I have thought and written about exponential growth, about the toll taken on caregivers, about parallels from history, about our need to connect.

Now I think about loss.

<><><>

We are in a period of time when numbers will become numbing in their recitation.

Perhaps they already are. Tens, hundreds, thousands, what does it even mean?

We can't connect to numbers.

We connect to their stories.

The stories behind them. The stories they tell.

◇◇◇

We will not truly fathom our losses for many lifetimes yet. Some of us never will.

I'm not a philosopher or a psychologist.

I'm just a human being.

When I think of loss, I think of the everyday gaps left behind.

The spaces in between that are so subtle yet devastating.

◇◇◇

There is a pair of shoes in a closet.

They were bought as a gift. They were used for running, and hiking, and for countless steps.

Those soles touched the dirt on Adirondack trails, the sand on Montauk beach, and the pavement on Madison Avenue.

They'll never be worn again.

◇◇◇

There is a pet dog, waiting.

He is a little dog, but he has an oversize personality.

He has known only one owner since he was a puppy.

The entirety of his life has been spent in unconditional love.

He will never see his owner again, and he won't understand why.

◇◇◇

There is a red car parked in a garage.

It is gathering dust, which is something it has never done before. Not like this.

It has been driven hundreds of thousands of miles. It has carried a man, and his family, faithfully.

It will be sold. Its stories will be forgotten.

◇◇◇

There is a sketchbook in a closet.

Its pages are filled with charcoal sketches. They are powerful, and fanciful, and beautiful.

There are stories behind every sketch. Moments in time.

There is one person who knows all the stories.

She will never get to tell them.

◇◇◇

There is a box of medals in a secret drawer.

They were given for bravery, for valor. The man who earned them never bragged. He kept them hidden.

But he would take them out now and then, and remember his band of brothers, and weep.

They will never be taken out again.

◇◇◇

There is a box of cereal on a shelf.

There's nothing particularly special about this cereal. It is sugary. It is artificially flavored. It has bright colors.

And it was a young man's favorite, since he was little.

He was the only one who liked it.

Now it is thrown away.

◇◇◇

No, we won't understand our collective losses. Not for many lifetimes. Perhaps never.

My vision blurs with tears as thoughts linger, and I hear numbers in a steady recitation.

I watch the raindrops streak upward on my windshield, as if racing one another to rejoin the sky.

No Normal

He'll never know exactly when he got infected with COVID-19. It's a thought that resurfaces now and then. A lingering loose end.

He does spend a lot of his time being exposed to it as he works in the ICUs, but he is meticulous with his PPE.

◇◇◇

It begins with a runny nose.

The runny nose is followed by chills.

He self-quarantines, just to be safe. By the time a cough is developing, he has tested positive.

◇◇◇

The shortness of breath comes on relatively rapidly.

He checks his oxygen levels at home and decides he needs to go to the hospital.

◇◇◇

Being admitted to a hospital he has worked at is a somewhat surreal experience.

So this is what it's like.

Everyone wearing their PPEs. Familiar, yet distant.

Like space travelers peering at him through the unforgiving void and the safety of their air locks.

◇◇◇

He reviews his own chest X-rays and lab data with the attending pulmonologist.

He feels confident he is going to get better. He's over 60, but he's fit, and he's in good hands.

He can't deny, though, that it's getting harder to breathe. He feels his respiratory rate climb.

◇◇◇

Have you ever thought about your breathing on a moment-by-moment basis?

If you haven't, consider yourself lucky.

To have to work to breathe, really work at it with every breath you take, is exhausting.

And terrifying.

He is transferred to the intensive care unit.

◇◇◇

In the ICU there is a strange tranquility.

The landscape isn't alien to him. He knows these machines, these people.

He hasn't been put on a ventilator, but he's getting close.

One day he sees his chest X-ray and has trouble identifying healthy lung tissue.

"God . . ."

◇◇◇

The attending pulmonologist talks to him, his face on a video screen.

Things aren't looking good. They're considering ECMO, but kidney function is worsening too.

He feels icy pangs of fear.

But he has things he needs to do now.

He suppresses the fear and calls his wife.

◇◇◇

He goes over things with her. Financial details, insurance details, passwords and codes, all the minutiae needed for a life stopped in mid-sentence.

She understands what he's saying. She's stoic, like him.

She takes notes quietly, as he takes short, quick breaths.

◇◇◇

He falls silent, and she is quiet too.

The truth is he's scared, but he's also tired.

He's been in the ICU for several days. He's tired of being out of breath.

So he doesn't speak now. He closes his eyes and listens to his wife tell him about their grandkids.

Later that night, he has hallucinations.

He dreams vividly that his grandkids are playing.

He savors these glimpses of his life before.

Of love.

The steady beeps of the monitors bring him back to reality. He watches the nurses move in their armor, and is grateful.

◇◇◇

The thought occurs to him repeatedly, as he feels the slow rush of air in and out of his lungs.

The irony isn't lost on him.

He is a pulmonologist, and all he can think about now is how he took every precious breath for granted.

He knows where this is going.

Dying breaths.

◇◇◇

Days pass, and he feels like he is in a strange purgatory. An in-between world, where he teeters on the edge of the precipice.

Intensive care, every day. Small steps.

One breath, then the next.

◇◇◇

Then one day he wakes up and notices that it's a little easier to breathe.

His oxygen saturation levels are better. They're able to wean his oxygen down slowly.

He is eventually moved out of the ICU to an intermediate unit.

He is on the road to recovery.

◇◇◇

The ordeal has caused him to lose a lot of weight and muscle mass.

He has to go to rehabilitation for several weeks.

Finally, he goes home.

About a month later, he is back at work, taking care of COVID patients in the ICU.

He tells his story to a wide-eyed nephrologist.

◇◇◇

I watch him, later in the day, intubating a crashing patient.

Only his eyes are visible beneath the masks and shield. His gaze is steady. Once again staring down the Monster.

I respect his courage.

I respect his skill.

Most of all I respect him for who he is.

Later I sit beside him.

I know he has gone through something I can't know.

We sit in silence.

Finally he speaks.

"You know the question people ask me the most?"

I shake my head.

"When are things going back to normal?" He shakes his head.

I say nothing.

◇◇◇

"There's going to be two groups of people. One group might have a normal again. The other? No normal, my friend. Just before and after."

I nod, thinking about what he's gone through. What so many people have gone through.

Before.

After.

And every breath in between.

Mondays and Fridays

Every day I see the same cook in the hospital cafeteria.

I say hello and ask him the same question.

"How's it going?"

He always smiles and shrugs. "Eh, not bad for a Monday."

Except he says "not bad for a Monday" every day of the week.

Finally I ask him about it.

◇◇◇

"Look, Doc, any day you gotta wake up early and go to work, heck, that's a Monday in my book."

"So, a workweek is five Mondays?"

"Yeah!" He laughs.

Another cook stands beside him. She shakes her head. "Don't listen to him, Doc."

I offer her a grin, as she continues.

◇◇◇

"I've been real sick in my life. I know how sick people are in this place. Every day isn't a Monday, it's a Friday, because every day is a blessing, and you look forward to the next one. For me, every day is a day I wasn't guaranteed. A second chance."

I nod, and smile.

◇◇◇

I'm still thinking about that conversation as I get on the elevator.

There are four of us in here. We each stand in one corner, saying nothing, face shields and masks on.

We all know where we are going.

We've been there before.

This place that haunts us.

◇◇◇

I talk to my friend, the intensivist, at our usual meeting place in the ICU dictation room.

"How's the COVID situation?"

"Bad. Intubated four people today. Trachs coming up for another four. It's . . . bad."

She rests her forehead on her palm as she talks to me.

Exhausted.

◇◇◇

She has finished rounding. Now she sits at her workstation and makes her day's phone calls, to all the family members who can't be there.

I listen.

I make my fair share of these calls too. They never get any easier.

Her voice is gentle. "I'm sorry."

Her gaze is far away.

◇◇◇

Later in the day I enter one of the COVID ICUs.

What was once foreign and chilling to witness has become cruelly routine.

The sight of humans on their bellies on ventilators, glimpsed through many layers of glass and plastic, doesn't affect me anymore.

Not like it used to.

◇◇◇

Every now and then I see something that jolts me. That reminds me of the stakes. That puts human beings into context.

But mostly my emotion has been stripped away.

I exist here and now in this netherworld, where we once were and where we are once again.

I hate this place.

◇◇◇

Our numbers are climbing inevitably upward. Thousands more will die, even as we are on the cusp of a vaccine rollout.

I think of a photo I saw once, of a soldier killed in World War I, just days before the armistice.

All this needless death, in the dusk.

<><><>

At the end of the day, I'm heading to the parking garage via the basement of the hospital.

As I walk down a hallway, I pass by a man pushing a stretcher. It is covered in a heavy embroidered black drape.

I know what it means.

I say a silent prayer.

God help us all.

Sitting in my car, I exhale deeply.

I look at my hands gripping the steering wheel, something I can control, knuckles turning white.

Was today a Monday or a Friday?

A blessing? Or just another damn day?

The Ghost on the Corner

There's a ghost on the corner of 3rd and Broadway.

I noticed him the other day as I made a left turn at the light.

He wasn't there a week ago.

He must be new.

Nobody I recognize, but then again, his face is blurry and indistinct.

I look at him now, and I drive past.

◇◇◇

Arriving at the hospital, I park my car.

More ghosts here, even in the parking lot.

Some of them stand beside empty cars and look into them wistfully, as if wishing for keys to unlock their escape.

I recognize some of these ghosts.

I look at them now, and I walk past.

◇◇◇

The hospital is busier than I can remember it being . . . ever.

The ER looks like a war zone, hallways filled, ambulances lining up outside.

"Don't they know we're on diversion?"

"Who knows, man, they came here anyways."

I grit my teeth and make sure my N95 is tight.

◇◇◇

The COVID wards are being reopened, again.

This time, however, it's different. There's no sense of imminent danger like there was before.

The feeling of fear has been replaced by a grim inevitability.

Return to work, fast as you can.

You are expendable.

You always were.

◇◇◇

It makes me think of World War I and trench warfare.

We keep digging these trenches to nowhere and convincing ourselves everything's okay, only to hear the whistle again and be given the order to charge.

And so we charge into no-man's-land, side by side.

Surge by surge.

◇◇◇

I get off the elevator at the ICU.

Nowhere in the hospital are there more ghosts than here.

They pace the hallways.

Angry at the way they died. Disbelieving. Disoriented at how fast it happened. Feeling cheated.

They all want something more.

More than this.

◇◇◇

COVID patients are short of breath, again. I'm looking at the same damn chest X-rays, again.

They tell me this is a milder variant.

What does that mean? "Milder"?

Can you please sit down and explain it to the ghost outside that room over there?

That it was only "mild"?

◇◇◇

Oh, I get it. I understand the stats and the low likelihood of serious illness.

I get all of that.

I just don't see it.

I see another full hospital.

I. Am. So. Sick. Of. This.

All that remains of me is raw exposed nerves and deadened scar tissue in equal measure.

◇◇◇

I don't understand why some events leave such a collective mark on our psyche, while others we're supposed to just let slip away.

1,000,000 people dead and counting.

We aren't equipped to grieve on that scale. But we can, we should, acknowledge it instead of pushing past it.

◇◇◇

That's all so many of these ghosts want.

Acknowledgment.

One of my last patients of the day is also my sickest.

This is a pattern I have seen many times before: lungs too ravaged to salvage, multi-organ failure, kidneys struggling to maintain their homeostasis.

◇◇◇

As I look at them through the glass door of their room, the plastic protective isolation sheets make their face blurry and indistinct.

I confer with the intensivist and the cardiologist.

We all agree, there's not much left to offer besides comfort.

The end is inevitable.

I write my note and leave before the family arrives. Normally I would stick around for this conversation, but today I leave it to the intensivist.

There is a gravity in the presence of death and dying that exerts a palpable force.

I can only be exposed to it for so long.

◇◇◇

As I walk along the ICU hallway, I notice that the ghosts are gone.

They tend to clear out when Death makes its way through, stopping outside its assigned room.

In a detached part of my mind I can hear the sobbing of a family in the consultation room.

Weeping in unison.

◇◇◇

Back in the elevator, I close my eyes and breathe deeply.

Almost everyone I see these days tells me I look tired.

Time off helps, but it's a temporary salve. My writing helps, again, only temporarily.

Gotta get to the root of it all.

Where the ghosts live.

I can't today.

$\diamond\!\diamond\!\diamond$

At the end of the day, I head back to the parking lot.

As I walk, I remember a conversation I had earlier in the day.

"Did you know that in some languages the words for 'tomorrow' and 'yesterday' are the same?"

Time is a circle.

We only perceive the direction of its flow.

$\diamond\!\diamond\!\diamond$

A time will come, after COVID, when our society will need us to rely on one another to do the right thing again.

There's a ghost on the corner of 3rd and Broadway.

I noticed him the other day as I turned at the light.

He wasn't there a week ago.

He won't be gone tomorrow.

The Red Car

There is a car in the hospital parking lot.

It is a faded red, covered with dust.

Other cars have parked and then left on either side of it, every day, but this car remains.

I pass by it, as I find parking, on my way in to work.

I know what it means.

◇◇◇

There was a time when it wasn't faded red, covered in dust. There was a time, decades ago now, when it was brand new.

"Ruby red metallic!"

The car salesman flashes a winning grin.

"Isn't she a beauty? And to think she could be all yours!"

The young man smiles.

◇◇◇

In the years to come, people will often ask the young man, Why did you choose the bright red? It doesn't seem to fit his personality.

He is quiet and withdrawn.

His answer is always the same. "It isn't red. It's ruby red. Got Dorothy home safe, it'll do for me."

◇◇◇

Many years later he will discover that the original novel, *The Wonderful Wizard of Oz*, made no mention of ruby slippers.

They were invented for the movie, to sparkle in new Technicolor.

But that's of no matter.

◇◇◇

He drives his beloved ruby red car everywhere.

Across town. Across the state. Across the country.

When he gets married, a JUST MARRIED banner is hung from the rear bumper.

When his wife goes into labor, that ruby red hot rod breaks every speed record in the state.

◇◇◇

With the passage of time, he has to make more practical decisions. But he can't bring himself to sell his car. It's been good to him.

He knows he's being silly.

It's just a machine.

But he's wept behind the steering wheel, and he's laughed, and it's kept his family safe.

◇◇◇

So he stores it in his garage. And every now and then, on a weekend, he tinkers with it.

Visiting an old friend.

One who never passed judgment on him. Who only served him faithfully.

His kids grow older. He grows older too.

Perhaps he should sell it, maybe it's time.

◇◇◇

It's his wife who convinces him to keep it.

"If it wasn't for that beautiful car, I would never have married you!"

He laughs, but then she says something true.

"It's not your car anymore. It's your friend. There's always room for friends."

He understands her wisdom.

◇◇◇

She dies unexpectedly, several years later, from cancer that had been lurking and managed to escape detection.

He has lost his true love and his best friend.

The raw depths of his grief threaten to submerge him, and for a time, they do.

And that's okay.

He'll be okay.

So now his favorite thing to do is take long drives in his ruby red hot rod. It has become old enough to be cool again.

Retro fever.

His kids want to move back home, but he assures them he's fine. Not to worry.

He finds happiness, and freedom, on the open highway.

◇◇◇

One day he wakes up with a strange pain in his chest. It makes his breath catch.

He thinks about calling 911, but it subsides.

Just to be safe, he decides to go to the local ER and get checked out.

He gets into his beloved car and turns the ignition for the last time.

◇◇◇

As he parks in the hospital parking lot, he feels strangely nervous. Perhaps he should call the kids. But he doesn't want to worry them.

He gets out of the car and notices a blemish on the hood. Spitting onto his palm, he wipes it clean.

It is an unassuming farewell.

He will die later that evening. His children don't understand. Why didn't he call them? The reports they're getting make no sense. Massive MI? Heart failure? Kidney failure?

Failure?

But he was so strong.

He was Dad. He is Dad.

They fly home that very night, numb.

◇◇◇

It will be several weeks before his daughter realizes their dad's beloved hot rod isn't in the garage after she unlocks it.

They had all assumed he dialed 911.

They didn't realize he drove himself to the ER.

Immediately, they make their way back to the hospital to search.

◇◇◇

There is a car in the hospital parking lot.

It is a faded red, covered with dust.

Other cars have parked and left on either side of it, every day, but this car remains.

I pass by it, as I find parking, on my way in to work.

I know what it means.

Sometimes I wonder.

How much gas is still in the tank? How many journeys were still planned or unplanned? Where did it go? Where was it going?

It was a beautiful car, once, I can see that.

As I drive past it, I pray for rain.

(For all the love we leave behind—ST, February 20, 2020.)

Bella

"My name is Dug. I have just met you, and I love you."

—Dug the dog, *Up* (2009)

◇◇◇

The hospital rooms can have a numbing sameness.

The same four walls. The same TV. The same bed. The same white sheets, meticulously tucked.

The same plastic toothbrushes in the same "hospitality kits."

Sterile. Efficient. Drab.

◇◇◇

Patients make little personalizations where they can.

A get well card on a side table. A blanket of their own. Photographs on a wall. A little speaker to connect to their phone and play music.

In this way, they say "I was here. I am here. And I am myself. Unique."

◇◇◇

To Bella, however, every room is unique already.

The moment a person is inside it, Bella's impossibly refined senses can detect their uniqueness. And in doing so, she can sense what they need from her intuitively.

Bella is a golden retriever.

And she is a healer.

◇◇◇

Every now and then Bella and her human best friend, Anne, make their rounds together through the hospital.

Patients can request to see Bella. And sometimes the nurses make suggestions too; patients who might benefit from Bella's unique brand of medicine.

Her love.

◇◇◇

The first room today is filled with grief.

Bella senses it as she enters and hears it in the quietness of Anne's voice.

Bella's tail doesn't wag briskly. She is subdued.

She rests her head on the side of the bed, and the sick human holds her and weeps.

Bella loves them.

◇◇◇

Eventually they move on, and in the hallway several of the nurses come to pet Bella.

She holds out her paw to "shake hands." She beams, and her tail thumps against the floor as she's petted.

She absorbs their love.

And she gives it back.

Bella loves them.

◇◇◇

A visit to see a child always makes Bella's day.

Their scent is unique to her. Innocent.

Of all the humans, she loves children the most. They bring a surge of protective warmth inside her.

They're always so happy to see her, eyes wide with wondrous joy.

Bella loves them.

◇◇◇

Sometimes the grief touches the children's rooms too.

Unbearably.

Sometimes Bella doesn't enter right away, but she lingers by the door. Seeking permission to step into this most difficult of places.

Sometimes the parents want her there. Sometimes not.

Bella loves them.

◇◇◇

An elderly patient is always happy to see her. He pets her lovingly and says, "You're a good dog, Bella. You remind me of my dog. She was a good dog too."

The old man is deeply alone, in ways that Bella can sense, but Anne can't.

She sits by his feet.

Bella loves him.

◇◇◇

The doctor walking briskly down the hall seems lost in his thoughts. His gaze is distant, and he almost runs into Anne and Bella before seeing them and laughing.

"Hey, Anne! Hey, Bella! How are the dynamic duo today?"

Bella can sense the friendship in his voice.

◇◇◇

The doctor reaches down to pet her, before washing his hands with the foamy disinfectant whose scent fills Bella's nostrils all day.

She beams up at him, hoping for a treat, but he has no packets of peanut butter to offer her.

Bella loves him all the same.

And I love her too.

The Invisible Woman

She's not sure when she became invisible.

She nods and smiles to the people she walks past, but rarely gets a response.

Sometimes she'll say hello just to test the limits a little. Sometimes she'll get a mumbled response. Sometimes they just look startled.

She moves on.

◇◇◇

Her workday began at 6:00 AM. She is a food service worker.

The kitchen is in the bowels of the hospital, a vast and complex operation that churns out hundreds of meals a day, designed to fit dozens of restrictions and allergies.

She helps make the trays, then delivers them.

◇◇◇

It sounds simple enough, but the responsibility is awesome.

When she was little, she once choked on a piece of carrot. She remembers how she felt, as her vision swam in front of her and the world grew dark.

Her dad saved her with the Heimlich maneuver.

She remembers.

And so she feels the weight of her responsibility.

One meal of the wrong consistency to a patient on aspiration precautions could be deadly.

One meal loaded in potassium to a dialysis patient.

Or sodium and heart failure.

She is always aware.

◇◇◇

The trays are loaded onto a large cart. Teams of food service workers leave the kitchen, each pushing a cart, and fan out around the hospital.

She pushes her cart down the numerous hallways, making her rounds.

She sees more inpatients every day than most of the doctors.

◇◇◇

She verifies each patient's name and matches it to the tray she then delivers.

On to the next one.

Next. Brisk.

But she's human too. Kind, caring, empathic.

She always pauses to say hello.

She really doesn't have time for conversation, but she makes the time to say hi.

◇◇◇

Many of the patients are asleep, many of them don't, or can't, respond to her.

But there are some who say hello, who seem grateful for a little bit of conversation.

The pressure of her work is constant, but a little bit of conversation is the least she can do.

◇◇◇

Doctors and nurses often talk in front of her like she isn't there.

She doesn't have a medical background, so a lot of what she overhears is a confusing jumble.

But as the years have gone by, she's been able to learn which words bring tears more often than others.

◇◇◇

She's not sure when she became invisible.

She nods and smiles to the people she walks past, but rarely gets a response.

Sometimes she'll say hello just to test the limits a little. Often she'll get a mumbled response or a cursory look.

It hurts, sometimes.

There's an elderly patient in a room, who's been there for a long while.

She has gotten to know him, a few minutes at a time, over the days and weeks.

Their brief conversations have ranged far and wide, spanning hopes and dreams.

He reminds her of her grandfather.

◇◇◇

He is always awake when she stops by. When she's a little late, he needles her good-naturedly. She laughs.

He does something few people do. He asks her how her day is going and genuinely wants to know.

As rough as her day may be, one person genuinely cares.

She smiles.

◇◇◇

One day she doesn't have a tray with his name on it. Her heart sinks, and as she delivers the trays, she glances in his room.

It's empty.

She suddenly feels a lump in her throat.

Caring often exacts a terrible price, too high for some.

She has always paid it willingly.

◇◇◇

Trying not to let the concern in her voice show, she casually asks one of the nurses what happened to the elderly man.

"He's doing better. He transferred to a rehab last night. Oh, hey . . . you're Meg, right?"

She nods, relief washing over her in great waves.

◇◇◇

"Here, he left this for you." The nurse hands her a note.

She unfolds the small little slip of paper.

His handwriting is spidery, but legible: "Thank you."

She smiles, folding the paper and putting it in her pocket, as she pushes her empty cart back to the elevator.

◇◇◇

Standing in the corner of the elevator, she smiles to herself as two doctors have an animated conversation, as if she isn't there.

The paper in her pocket brings a deep and unexpected happiness.

She wasn't sure when she became invisible.

But today she cherishes being seen.

◇◇◇

(Thanks to the numerous food service workers I spoke to in multiple hospitals, their chefs, managers, and all the support staff.

The word "hero" is used a lot these days, appropriately.

This is for all the "invisible" everyday heroes. Thank you.

We see you.)

COVID-19, 2060

It isn't easy being 80 years old.

Things don't work like they used to. People don't treat you like they used to.

I'm standing before the shower in my hotel room.

"Temperature?" a voice asks me.

"Warm, but not too hot," I answer.

The shower starts, the water's perfect.

◇◇◇

Of course, I remember a time when things were different.

In my day, you had a hot water knob and a cold water knob and you had to experiment until the water temperature was just right.

My grandkids laugh when I tell them.

I'm a relic.

That's why I'm here.

◇◇◇

I finish showering and let the machines "flash-dry" me. I imagine this is what it feels like to be microwaved. Another device that's no longer around.

Putting on my suit, I tie my tie myself.

The cyborg concierge could do it, but I want to do at least this one thing.

◇◇◇

I leave my room and make my way to the elevators.

It wasn't my idea to attend this conference. An acquaintance of mine had reached out to me. An opportunity to catch up with old friends, he said.

I am to be "a link to the past."

A doctor who was there, to bear witness.

◇◇◇

The elevator is nearly silent as it whisks me down.

I look at my reflection in the mirrored doors. It's strange, I still don't quite recognize myself.

I know I'm 80. I'm not a young man.

But my mind doesn't feel the passage of years, not the way my body has.

◇◇◇

The doors slide open, and I step into the main lobby.

The banner is large, covering the main entrance archway.
COVID-19: ECHOES FROM THE PAST, 2060

People smile at me as I slowly make my way. I nod and smile in return.

◇◇◇

Nowadays, we are all wearing masks, protections made invisible by nanotechnology, see-through and almost impossible to feel.

◇◇◇

The only way you know someone is wearing one is the green light on their ID badge. If you're not wearing one at this conference, you get a flashing red light and a quick visit from a detox team.

◇◇◇

I enter the main lecture hall.
There is an eerie silence. Of course, I'm one of the few people attending in person.

Most people don't risk crowds anymore. They haven't for decades.

I make my way to an empty seat on the stage and sit down.

The moderator welcomes me.

◇◇◇

People want to know what it was like. I understand that.

Since COVID-19 there have been several others: HantaVM-26. COVID-35. FluVAR-59.

But people want to know about the "original." After all, our original mistakes are what changed everything.

Original sins.

As I look out from the stage, a sea of faces on video screens looks back at me.

How do I explain something called "Twitter" to them? How do they grasp "MedTwitter"? Those bonds we formed so long ago?

How do you explain "social media" to a society that IS media?

◇◇◇

The first lecturer is presenting.

There are graphs I've seen a thousand times.

The so-called American Aberrancy.

It's hard to describe to people nowadays what that mindset was like.

Global warming has destroyed most of our nationalistic tendencies.

We survive together.

◇◇◇

I remember when I was younger, meeting survivors of World War II. Trying to imagine their reality then, when the outcome of the war wasn't known.

I suppose that's how the audience sees me now. Someone who witnessed a great uncertainty.

And the best of us.

And the worst.

◇◇◇

My turn comes. I walk to the podium and I begin to speak.

I wrote down notes on cards. Archaic I know, but I like the way they feel.

I introduce myself, and try to paint a picture of the world before the virus.

My role is not to be an expert, but to be a living memory.

◇◇◇

I describe those first few news broadcasts. The denial that ran rampant. The confusion. The obfuscation. The masks and the anti-masks.

The fear.

Names that have become as well known as Normandy and Dunkirk: Wuhan and Bergamo.

The data and the disinformation.

◇◇◇

I know the vast majority of what I say sounds too bizarre to be true.

People questioning masks? Questioning distancing? Reopening despite the data?

Perhaps this is what Semmelweis or Lister might have felt were they to lecture a modern medical school class on hygiene.

◇◇◇

I finish my remarks on a note of hope. I describe the vaccines and therapies that brought us out of the darkness and helped to mitigate the subsequent waves.

I describe the investment in our healthcare systems and the massive societal overhauls as change finally came.

◇◇◇

My talk ends with the final global and American casualty figures for COVID-19 being projected on the screen behind me.

I look away.

I've never been able to look at those numbers without my eyes filling with tears and my heart sinking.

It didn't have to be that way.

◇◇◇

Afterward I'm making my way back to the elevators.

A young woman walks up to greet me.

She tells me her name and says she is a medical student and wanted to ask me a question, but not in front of everyone.

I smile and say hello. It's nice to talk to a person in the flesh.

◇◇◇

"You said you lost people you knew."

159

I nod. "Almost everyone did, in the end. Everyone knew someone."

"Did you lose something too? A part of you . . ."

I know what she's asking. We rarely discuss it.

Some scars never leave you.

You have to heal.

I smile and say nothing.

The Hand-Holder

There once was an oath that all doctors had to take. Something about doing the right thing and trying not to hurt anyone.

That was long ago, in the 21st century, before the machines. My great-grandfather took that oath.

Machines don't need oaths.

But I'm still human.

◇◇◇

The first thing that hits me is the smell. Coming to the Reach is always a stark reminder of just how impoverished some of us are.

Progress always leaves people behind. The question is who gets to choose who gets left behind and who rises.

I'm here to make a house call.

◇◇◇

I'm a physician, although in the 22nd century that phrase has lost most of its meaning.

We always thought people would want the human touch in healing.

But once machines were hitting 100% in their diagnostic accuracy and gene splicing and nanotech were viable, it was over.

◇◇◇

MD now stands for Medical Device, and refers to any of the hundreds of cyborg med-techs on the market.

Immortality is in your grasp if you can afford it.

Human physicians never see patients now. They just sit in control rooms, overseeing armies of med-techs.

Except me.

◇◇◇

Me and a few others like me are the last of a dying breed.

We offer medicine to those who can't afford an MD. Our society corporatized medicine long ago except for us few, making our last stand.

Derisively, our colleagues in the rich cities call us "hand-holders."

◇◇◇

"Hand-holders" because we don't have the tech to fix most problems. Not like they do.

But we still have skills, from a time long before the first machines performed their first solo surgeries.

So here I am, in the sprawling slums on the edge of the City known as the Reach.

◇◇◇

My nano-mask is filtering the air I breath, invisible over my face, and yet it can't get rid of the stench.

The smell of rot and decay hits me like a sledgehammer. The synthetic and sanitized City doesn't have smells like these.

I walk alone, except for Bernie beside me.

◇◇◇

MD-BRN1E786, or Bernie for short, is a decommissioned second-generation med-tech cyborg, virtually obsolete.

I got him on the black market. He provides some medical help and, more important, security.

There are many antimedicine cults out there, and most are violent.

◇◇◇

We walk together, in silence, Bernie's motors whirring quietly as he takes one plodding step after another beside me.

He's painted white and red, with MED-TECH stenciled helpfully across his chest.

"Almost there," I say out loud.

"Yes, 132 meters." Bernie's voice is chirpy.

◇◇◇

The dwelling we enter is a ramshackle affair, typical of the Reach. With flimsy walls leaning against each other and a dingy bulb swaying, lighting everything in a sickly glow.

The patient is a young girl, dressed in rags stitched together, lying motionless on the floor.

◇◇◇

Her father is kneeling beside her and looks up at me with a hollow gaze, bereft of hope.

I know better than to ask where the mother is. This is the Reach, after all. If you aren't present, you're in the past.

I kneel down and touch the girl's forehead. She's burning up.

◇◇◇

A quick glance at the floor next to her reveals empty bottles of "medicine." Most of them are scams, or diluted so much they're practically useless. Snake-oil salesmen are rampant in the Reach, preying on the vulnerable.

This girl is dying.

I take out my instruments.

◇◇◇

My great-grandfather was a physician, a long time ago. When medicine was still practiced by humans. He was a kidney doctor, an idea that seems quaint now.

I don't really know much about him, but I have his stethoscope, passed down to me. A relic.

I press it to the girl.

◇◇◇

Through the earpieces, I hear the crackling of fluid in the lungs. The thundering of her heart driven to a fury by her fevers and dilating vasculature.

A raging storm.

Bernie leans over her, next to me, his voice unreasonably cheerful. "Alert! Impending systems collapse!"

◇◇◇

My options are limited. I'm a hand-holder, after all. But I retrofitted Bernie a few months ago. It's risky, but I think he's the only chance the girl has.

I take her father aside and explain.

His face shows no emotion.

I understand.

How much more can one heart break?

◇◇◇

I enter the authorization codes on Bernie's interface, and leave the dwelling with the father, to give the cyborg space to initiate his "OR Protocol."

There's a brief flash of flickering blue light as Bernie sterilizes the room.

As he leans over the girl, I close the door.

◇◇◇

I stand outside the dwelling with the girl's father, breathing in the heavy smog, saying nothing.

He looks down at his feet, silent.

I want to ask him his story. How did he end up here? Was he born into this, like most of us, the end result of an unbalanced equation?

◇◇◇

As I'm lost in my thoughts, I feel a small tug on my heavy traveling cloak.

Glancing down, I see a child squatting in the dust by my feet. He says nothing, but holds his hands up, cupped together.

I have nothing to give him.

With his each breath I see his emaciated ribs.

◇◇◇

I know in the City, everyone has healthcare, and everyone has food.

I could try to take him to the City, beg for help. But those gates were closed to him the day he was born a "natural" birth, without the genetic coding that would gift him entrance.

"I'm sorry," I say.

◇◇◇

The child looks up at me one last time, then vanishes into the dark night.

To join the many faces I haven't helped, that gaze upon me in silent condemnation every time I close my eyes.

Hand-holder, they say, why didn't you hold our hands?

"I'm sorry," I say, over and over.

The hours pass. Finally the father speaks. "Is she gonna make it?"

I sigh. "She's in better hands with the med-tech than with me."

He nods, then gestures to a tiny disc I wear as a pendant around my neck.

"What's that?"

"It's a codex. It's called the Hippocratic oath."

◇◇◇

"What's the Hippocratic oath?"

"I don't know, it belonged to my great-grandfather. The file's damaged, I can't read it."

"So why do you keep it?"

"Good luck, I guess."

Bernie emerges from the house. Cheerful as always, he chirps, "Procedure success! Patient resting."

◇◇◇

A light enters the father's eyes. For the first time, he smiles. "Thank you. I don't have much to pay you. But I can fix that codex."

I smile in return, taking off the pendant and handing it to him. "Thank you."

The truth is, no hand-holder ever gets paid, not with money.

The father disappears into his home, and I'm left running Bernie's post-op analytics.

After a few minutes, the father steps out again, handing me my codex back.

"It wasn't broken, just scratched."

I nod. "Thanks."

Then I read it for the first time.

The Hippocratic oath.

◇◇◇

There once was an oath that all doctors had to take.

An oath, reaching across the centuries, reminding me.

Kindling a fire.

Why we go to those who suffer, and why we hold their hands.

I walk with Bernie, away from the Reach, and into the lonely darkness of the endless night.

PART V

Endings

The Shoreless Ocean: Life Advice to Students and Learners

To med students, and students of all fields:

Time takes many things away from you as it passes.

Life is often a difficult lesson in letting go.

But time also gives you one gift: a precious, powerful gift.

A gift that can alter your very reality.

The gift of perspective.

So here's mine.

◇◇◇

I graduated from medical school in 2004, almost twenty years ago.

Reading people's anxious tweets about med school took me back.

That constant feeling that it's all out of your hands, no matter how hard you try.

The gnawing uncertainty.

The imposter syndrome.

The stress.

Let me just say something up front, none of what I'm about to say is supposed to let medical education off the hook.

Because, let's face it, there's plenty that needs to be fixed in medical education. There was plenty twenty years ago. There is plenty now.

It's profoundly dysfunctional.

◇◇◇

And also none of what I'm about to say necessarily applies to everyone.

I can only speak to my own personal experiences and my own personal thoughts.

So if you get the urge to say "Hey, you're wrong, I didn't experience that," I totally agree with you.
You're right.

◇◇◇

The path to medicine requires many things. Discipline, work, patience, delayed gratification.

There's this tendency to look at medicine as the mountaintop.

It's this distant peak you're striving toward, wreathed in clouds.

And just like mountain climbing, it's perilous.

◇◇◇

Your oxygen can run low, the weather can change, handholds that seem sure can suddenly turn treacherous, and even with teamwork you can lose people along the way.

You can lose yourself along the way.

What do I realize looking back on it now?

It was never a mountain at all.

◇◇◇

Medicine is a shoreless ocean.

It begins long before you ever step foot in a medical school, and it keeps going long after you think you'll pass some final hurdle.

It's not about ascending to some great heights.

It's about learning your own depths, and how to swim together with others.

◇◇◇

I know these are just analogics, so here are some more thoughts.

In twenty years I've never cared where someone went to med school, or did their residency, or whether they're an IMG, or whether they're a DO or MD.

I care about what kind of a doctor they are, who they've become.

◇◇◇

The fact that their education tells me nothing about their skills as a doctor should tell you something.

It isn't that they conquered some distant mountain peak.

They're in the same ocean as I am, as we all are.

All that matters is what kind of a doctor it makes them.

There will be things that tend to happen. You will do worse than you thought on a test. You will do poorly and have bad days.

Some days you'll swear the entire floor saw how bad you did something, and everyone laughed.

Nobody will remember, twenty years from now.

◇◇◇

And while you've been worrying about a million different things, and facing a million different hurdles, something else has been happening.

Something amazing.

You're becoming a doctor.

It started long before med school, when you started becoming your own person.

◇◇◇

It'll continue long after med school is over, because you never stop swimming, and the ocean is endless.

Because the ocean isn't just medicine, is it? It's knowledge. It's humanity. It's life.

There will always be another exam. Another test, another trial.

That's life.

◇◇◇

Use the ocean. Strengthen your lungs, learn to breathe deeply. Learn to go with the currents, and learn to fight them.

Learn to help one another, because we all tire, inevitably.

And know that you are essential, and you belong here, and you aren't alone.

You're never alone.

◇◇◇

Yes, there are sharks in the ocean. Yes, there are monsters in the deep.

Yes, it's possible to drown in this ocean.

The system isn't perfect. It wasn't perfect twenty years ago. It needs to measure better things. It needs to teach better things.

◇◇◇

I'm no medical education expert. I can't pinpoint what needs to change. I just know that it needs to.

You might argue that you can't change an ocean.

Maybe.

But you can swim faster, and stronger.

You can build better boats.

◇◇◇

No matter where you go, what doors open or close, you'll be okay.

Remember why you're here.

Remember who you are.

You belong. You always did.

There are people you don't even know exist, who will someday be counting on you.

Author's Note

I was lucky to find a circle of friends and supporters on Twitter. Twitter can sometimes feel like a raging river, and it takes an act of courage even to dip your toe in the water. There are thousands of tweets every second, half a billion tweets every day. Without an audience, tweeting can sometimes feel like screaming into the void.

But once people found me, I was struck by their willingness to support my writing. Total strangers sent me messages of thanks. Shared their own stories of life, love, and loss. My stories started being shared and then re-shared. Soon I was writing for an audience I had never imagined having. It was a tremendous affirmation, and a blessing I was lucky to get.

Going viral is strangely disorienting. Everything feels surreal, and at first the approval is exhilarating, but also daunting and humbling. A strong dose of imposter syndrome has always followed me. I remain convinced as of the time of my writing these words that my writing is not particularly exceptional, nor is it memorable. But my words do seem to resonate with people, and for this I am grateful.

Cherish your stories.

Listen to one another's.

It's been an amazing journey writing this book.

Acknowledgments

The short stories in this book concern my journey into medicine: some of the mentors who guided me, the patients who taught me, and the family in whose footsteps I follow.

In medicine, every patient presents with a story. "Once upon a time I was well and then . . ." The narrative, the story, is at the beating heart of medicine. It is through stories that we communicate, that we strive to understand, that we begin to empathize and perhaps to heal.

This project could not have come to fruition without the kindness and support of thousands of people on Twitter who followed me before I had anything to show for myself. Who believed in me while I was still finding my voice. I am deeply indebted to them.

And to my colleagues and my friends, who show me every day what it means to be wonderful and caring human beings. And Lisa Sharkey with HarperCollins, who gave me the great gift of believing in my vision. And Adenike Olanrewaju, who helped me mold the project into its final form with her unique blend of wisdom and patience.

And, of course, my wife and my family. They gave me all the love, and from there the words flowed.

About the Author

SAYED TABATABAI is a nephrologist and writer. He shares most of his work with his large audience on Twitter on his handle @The RealDoctorT, and his writing has appeared in *Medium*, *Physicians Weekly*, the *Wall Street Journal*, and on NPR. He lives in San Antonio.